Praise for Against th

"Arno and Feiden ably depict the anger and frustration that swelled up to challenge the traditional pace of research and drug approval policy. . . . The authors write with a breeziness accessible to the general public."   —*Science*

"Lively and compelling throughout. . . . This book will be of great interest to a broad array of readers."—June E. Osborn, M.D., Dean, University of Michigan School of Public Health, and Chair, National Commission on AIDS

"This intensely researched chronicle puts it all into perspective. A must read!"—Donald I. Abrams, M.D., Associate Professor, University of California, San Francisco

"*Against the Odds* compellingly illustrates how the drug approval process has wreaked havoc on delivery of care to HIV-infected people."   —*Modern Healthcare*

"Inspiring documentation showing that motivated and organized patients can make a difference."   —*Kirkus Reviews*

"An incisive view of how health activism has become an invaluable tool."   —*Publishers Weekly*

"A hard-hitting, superbly written analysis of an area of vital importance to all Americans."—Philip R. Lee, M.D., Director, Institute for Health Policy Studies, University of California, San Francisco

"Peter Arno and Karyn Feiden explain with wisdom, eloquence and passion this extraordinary story as well as its significance for every American."—Thomas B. Stoddard, former executive director, Lambda Legal Defense and Education Fund

"An important history of courageous people who, in a fight for their lives, have made history."—David Barr, Assistant Director of Policy, Gay Men's Health Crisis

"Brilliant. . . . Everyone who is concerned with AIDS, as patient, health professional, decision-maker, taxpayer or voter, should read this book."—Victor W. Sidel, M.D., Distinguished University Professor of Social Medicine, Montefiore Medical Center, Albert Einstein College of Medicine

"A story of heroism and foolishness that cries out to be told. A look at the unbridled greed, the human consequences of professional pride, the indifference of federal bureaucrats and the catastrophic financial and physiological burdens that resulted in AIDS patients taking matters into their own hands."—Abbey S. Meyers, Executive Director, National Organization for Rare Disorders

"The best history yet of institutional failure and community response in AIDS treatment, research, and access—an important book for improving future medical research."—John S. James, Editor and Publisher, *AIDS Treatment News*

"Arno and Feiden show how the absence of Federal leadership and commitment has compounded the damage the AIDS virus has inflicted and how ordinary citizens have improved the social structure. Should be mandatory reading."—Donald P. Francis, M.D., D.Sc., formerly, Centers for Disease Control

"A dramatic and poignant examination of the decade-long search for a cure and treatment for AIDS."   —*Rocky Mountain News*

"Eminently worthwhile, for those whose lives have been directly touched by AIDS as well as for those simply wishing to learn more about this horrifying plague."   —*Cleveland Plain Dealer*

AGAINST THE ODDS

AGAINST THE ODDS

The Story of AIDS Drug Development, Politics and Profits

PETER S. ARNO

AND

KARYN L. FEIDEN

HarperPerennial

A Division of HarperCollinsPublishers

First HarperPerennial edition published 1993.

Designed by Irving Perkins Associates

The Library of Congress has catalogued the hardcover edition as follows:

Arno, Peter S., 1954–
    Against the odds: the story of AIDS drug development, politics and profits / Peter S. Arno and Karyn L. Feiden. — 1st ed.
      p. cm.
    Includes bibliographical references and index.
    ISBN 0-06-018309-8 (cloth)
    1. AIDS (Disease)—Government policy—United States.   2. AIDS (Disease)—Chemotherapy.   3. Clinical drug trials—Government policy—United States.   I. Feiden, Karyn L.   II. Title.
RA644.A25A76   1992
362.1'969792—dc20   90-55947

ISBN 0-06-092359-8 (pbk.)

93 94 95 96 97 CC/HC 10 9 8 7 6 5 4 3 2 1

*In memory of John Griggs, our friend and colleague,
and so many others who fought against the odds
with courage, conviction, and dignity.*

"I've seen the statistics and, as you say, they're most perturbing."

"They're more than perturbing; they're conclusive."

"I'll ask government for orders. . . ."

"Orders!" he said scornfully. "When what's needed is imagination."

—Albert Camus, *The Plague*

CONTENTS

ACKNOWLEDGMENTS

A BOOK such as this cannot be researched, written, and published without a huge supporting cast. Any errors of fact or interpretation are strictly our own, but we trust that all the help we received has kept those to a minimum.

In particular, we would like to acknowledge the American Foundation for AIDS Research, which provided some support for this project, and the Department of Epidemiology and Social Medicine at Montefiore Medical Center and Albert Einstein College of Medicine, headed by Michael Alderman, which provided a congenial and supportive atmosphere in which to research and write this book. Ernie Drucker, Steve Martin, John Arras, and Bob Klein, all colleagues in the department, generously read and commented on various portions of the manuscript and Bob was especially helpful in clarifying a number of complex scientific issues.

Several others also read drafts of *Against the Odds* and shared their insights and concerns with us; their comments improved this book immeasurably. Thanks to David Barr, Gay Men's Health Crisis; Ron Bayer, Columbia School of Public Health; Martin Delaney, Project Inform; Don Francis, Centers for Disease Control; Jesse Green, New York University Medical Center; Peggy Hamburg, New York City Health Department; Bob Hughes, Robert Wood Johnson Foundation; Phjl Lee, University of California, San Francisco; Carol Levine, Citizens Commission on AIDS; Abbey Meyers, National Organization for Rare Disorders; Gerald Oppenheimer, Brooklyn College; June Osborn, University of Michigan School of Public Health; Vic Sidel, Montefiore Medical Center; Merv Silverman, American Foundation for AIDS Research; Thomas Stoddard, formerly with Lambda Legal Defense and Education Fund; and Tim Westmoreland, Subcommittee on Health and the Environment, U.S. Congress.

Some of the issues discussed in *Against the Odds* are complex and sensitive and we would not have been confident about our material without regular access to some of the most knowledgeable people in the field. The expertise and generosity of Brian Wolfman, an attorney with Public Citizen, and Michael Davis, a law professor at Cleveland State University, made it possible for us to tackle the issue of the AZT patent in all its arcane detail. In addition we would like to thank Sid Wolfe and David Vladeck, also of Public Citizen, who successfully challenged the Public Health Service's initial refusal to provide us access to public documents under the Freedom of Information Act.

Derek Hodel, who runs the PWA Health Group, was always helpful in providing us with hard-to-obtain documents and Patsy Fleming, a top aide to Congressman Ted Weiss, frequently shared her insider's perspective about AIDS politics on Capitol Hill. Gerald Friedland, formerly at Montefiore and now at Yale, helped with insightful comments about the clinical trials process.

Many sources within the Food and Drug Administration, the National Institute of Allergy and Infectious Diseases, and the National Cancer Institute were also extremely cooperative in meeting our numerous requests for information.

Additional thanks go to the dozens of other people who consented to be interviewed; a complete list is provided in the back of this book.

Tom Miller, our editor at HarperCollins, had a commitment to this project that was rare, and his hands-on editorial approach, with the help of Jim Hornfischer, helped give the book its coherence. Our agent, Barbara Lowenstein of Lowenstein Associates, was enthusiastic, demanding, and supportive, as always.

Lewis Clayton was, as always, extremely generous in his moral and legal support. Lesley Sussman's wit, wisdom, and journalistic insights helped broaden the appeal of this book, and his willingness to read numerous drafts went well beyond the call of duty. Karen Bonuck was a creative researcher who tirelessly chased down obscure facts, tracked sources, made endless telephone calls, and, throughout it all, showed extraordinary patience and good humor. Vernon Bluette, the librarian at Montefiore Medical Center, and Renée Trell, who provided preliminary research assistance, also played crucial roles in digging up needed information. Margie Graulau's secretarial services and her capacity to read copy that was often upside-down, sideways, or backwards were remarkable.

Finally, we have personal acknowledgments that can never be adequately expressed. As months dragged by and we struggled to finish this project, we wondered whether life would ever return to normal. Throughout, those we love offered their encouragement, support, patience, and humor. Peter's wife, Iris Hiskey Arno, also brought her editorial talents and a fresh outlook to this manuscript. To Iris, their two sons, Max and Zachary, and to Karyn's devoted partner, David Elsasser, we offer our gratitude and our love.

INTRODUCTION

Against the Odds is the product of three years of research and writing, although the book had its true genesis much earlier. Almost since the beginning of the AIDS epidemic, both of us have observed and commented on the nation's failures to address AIDS appropriately—Peter, in his capacity as a health economist and policy analyst, Karyn as a writer specializing in issues of public health. Back in 1986 we scrutinized the Reagan Administration's early responses and, in a journal article, concluded that "the picture that emerges from the analysis of the federal response to AIDS is of a nation still ill-prepared to respond to a crisis, an Administration too blinded by its own ideology to know when to reorder its priorities, and a fragmented health-care system unable to distribute the financial burden of catastrophic illness equitably."

Those facts have unfortunately changed little since then, and our concerns—both personal and political—have grown. The failures of the recent past reflect deeply ingrained structural problems. In stark contrast to almost every other developed nation, the United States does not guarantee decent health care as a basic human right. With AIDS, as with other diseases, this means poor people and minorities do not have adequate access to medical treatment or promising new therapies. Society's continued intolerance of homosexuality, its institutionalized racism, and the dominance of corporate influence all contributed to the hammerlock that precluded a timely response to the AIDS epidemic. And the absence of bold leadership—in fact, of *any* leadership—from the White House for more than a decade remains unforgivable.

Like so many others, we have lost friends and colleagues to AIDS. The desire to come to grips with the tragedy of this epidemic was part of our motivation for writing this book. We were also driven by the conviction that as a paradigm mirroring the multiple failures of the nation's health-care system—ranging from extortionate drug-pricing practices to the absence of quality care for the disenfranchised—the epidemic has much to teach us. Finally, we were inspired by the extraordinary display of activist solidarity and patient empowerment that spurred radical changes in drug development and distribution. The courageous actions of these people are a symbol of hope to those seeking progressive social change. Let them also be a warning to those who defend the status quo and the business-as-usual mentality that still pervades the nation's thinking about AIDS.

The issues surrounding AIDS drug development are complex, and the struggle has rarely been one between good guys and bad. Over the past decade many individuals in positions of authority risked their lives and careers to make a difference. Sadly, there have been others who could have done more for people with AIDS, but did not. Had some substituted a broader vision for scientific rigidity, had others put compassion above profit, some of the suffering would have been eased.

In this book we have taken many in the public health establishment to task, yet we have no particular ax to grind. To the contrary, both of us work closely with many in the same agencies that we have criticized. We have tried to present a balanced picture of what happened in AIDS drug development, focusing on the years between the approval of AZT in March 1987 and the approval of ddI four and a half years later, in October 1991. These were extraordinary years—years when terminally ill patients found the strength to awaken bureaucrats and scientists to their needs, and to pave the way for a new era of health activism.

CAST OF CHARACTERS

Donald Abrams, M.D., associate professor of clinical medicine, University of California, San Francisco; executive director, County Community Consortium, San Francisco, Calif.

David Barr, attorney, Lambda Legal Defense, Gay Men's Health Crisis, and ACT UP, New York, N.Y.

Bernard Bihari, M.D., former medical director, Community Research Initiative, New York, N.Y.

Sam Broder, M.D., director, National Cancer Institute, Bethesda, Md.

Michael Callen, long-term AIDS survivor and activist; co-founder, Community Research Initiative, New York, N.Y.

Ellen Cooper, M.D., former director, Antivirals Division, Food and Drug Administration, Rockville, Md.

James Corti, master smuggler, AIDS drug underground, Los Angeles, Calif.

Michael Davis, law professor, Cleveland State University College of Law; expert on U.S. patent law, Cleveland, Ohio.

Martin Delaney, executive director, Project Inform, San Francisco, Calif.

Jim Eigo, member, AIDS Treatment and Data Committee, ACT UP, New York, N.Y.

Anthony Fauci, M.D., director, National Institute of Allergy and Infectious Diseases, Bethesda, Md.

Margaret Fischl, M.D., Department of Medicine, University of Miami School of Medicine, Miami, Fla.

James Foster, consultant to Lyphomed; member, San Francisco Health Commission, San Francisco, Calif. Now deceased.

T. E. Haigler, former president, Burroughs Wellcome Company, Research Triangle, N.C.

Mark Harrington, member, AIDS Treatment and Data Committee, ACT UP, New York, N.Y.

Derek Hodel, executive director, PWA Health Group, New York, N.Y.

Daniel Hoth, M.D., director, Division of AIDS, National Institute of Allergy and Infectious Diseases, Bethesda, Md.

John James, editor, *AIDS Treatment News*, San Francisco, Calif.

David A. Kessler, M.D., commissioner, Food and Drug Administration, Rockville, Md.

Gina Kolata, reporter, *New York Times.*

Larry Kramer, co-founder, Gay Men's Health Crisis; co-founder, ACT UP, New York, N.Y.

Mathilde Krim, Ph.D., founding chairperson, American Foundation for AIDS Research, New York, N.Y.

Jeff Levi, director, Government Affairs, AIDS Action Council, Washington, D.C.; former executive director, National Gay and Lesbian Task Force.

Jay Lipner, attorney and activist, New York, N.Y. Now deceased.

Jean McGuire, former director, AIDS Action Council, Washington, D.C.

Abbey Meyers, executive director, National Organization of Rare Disorders, New Fairfield, Conn.

Hiroaki Mitsuya, M.D., Ph.D., chief, Experimental Retrovirology Section, Medicine Branch, National Cancer Institute, Bethesda, Md.

Peter Staley, member, AIDS Treatment and Data Committee, ACT UP, New York, N.Y.

Brian Tambi, president and chief executive officer, Fujisawa Pharmaceutical Company; former senior vice-president, Lyphomed, Rosemont, Ill.

Paul Volberding, M.D., chief, AIDS Program and Clinical Oncology, San Francisco General Hospital, San Francisco, Calif.

Henry Waxman, member of Congress; chairman, Subcommittee on Health and the Environment of the Committee on Energy and Commerce, United States House of Representatives, Washington, D.C.

Ted Weiss, member of Congress; chairman, Human Resources and Intergovernmental Relations Subcommittee of the Committee on Government Operations, United States House of Representatives, Washington, D.C.

Frank Young, M.D., former commissioner, Food and Drug Administration, Rockville, Md.

AGAINST THE ODDS

1

UNLIKELY HEROES

❖

Si monumentum requiris, circumspice.
If you seek a monument, look about you.

—Epitaph on CHRISTOPHER
WREN's tomb,
St. Paul's Cathedral, London

THIS IS A STORY of inspiration and despair, of hope and luck run out. The story begins in the 1980s, when a modern-day plague began to take its toll. And the story is true.

From the Castro District of San Francisco to the streets of Greenwich Village, AIDS first struck with brutal force in gay communities across America. Then it blazed a trail of death in Jersey City and the South Bronx, in East Los Angeles and Miami's Liberty Hill—poor and largely minority neighborhoods where shattered families, poor health, and drug abuse were already endemic. Now it has spread to small towns and cities across America, where denial is still common and necessary medical and social services are sparse.

Ten years have passed and the vicious epidemic has not relented. There is no cure, and few effective treatments exist. More than 200,000 Americans have succumbed to the illness and at least one million more are probably infected with the AIDS virus. Unless a spectacular scientific breakthrough comes soon, most of these people will be dead before the new millennium.

1

Yet from the depths of such despair, a movement has been born; heroes have emerged.

Many of the key players had AIDS themselves. Others responded to needs in their communities and to personal tragedies. Together, these people have empowered themselves in ways never seen before in the health-care arena. Confronted by governmental apathy and corporate neglect, they refused to remain passive or to be victimized. Instead, they stood on the shoulders of the social revolutions that came before—the civil rights struggle, the peace movement, the women's movement, and the drive for gay rights—and pursued one agenda with singleminded determination: treatments that might save lives.

Some spoke quietly, concentrating their efforts on behind-the-scenes strategies to prod and push the sluggish bureaucracy. As the toll of AIDS deaths mounted, others took to the streets demanding an end to society's indifference.

Their insistent voices began to be heard. Their radical demands meshed with conservative voices in the pharmaceutical industry and with ideologues who favored loosening the federal regulatory leash. Their interplay has helped transform the way in which drugs are developed and regulated in the United States.

In the 1970s, gay men began to express their sexual identity openly. Many left small towns to carve out gay ghettos in New York City, San Francisco, Los Angeles, Miami, and other urban enclaves where attitudes were more open. A new era in sexual politics was launched.

Living in predominantly gay communities for the first time, they were freed from the shackles of repression, and many previous behavioral norms suddenly seemed old-fashioned and irrelevant. The politics of gay liberation became linked with free sexuality. In certain circles it became commonplace to have dozens of sexual partners in a single night. Large numbers of men found fast and anonymous pleasure at the bathhouses and the barrooms, on abandoned docks and park benches. As breeding grounds for infection, such places were ideal. But no one gave much thought to that possibility. Certainly not healthy young adults, who had been vaccinated against polio, the last terrible infectious disease to strike Americans. Their confidence in the miracles of Western medicine was widely shared—

the prospect of a new epidemic in an industrialized nation seemed remote.

Eventually a wave of sexually transmitted diseases shook that confidence. Gonorrhea, syphilis, trichomoniasis, herpes, and chlamydia spread through large segments of the gay community. Gastrointestinal parasites like amebiasis, giardiasis, and shigellosis became commonplace, and hepatitis B reached epidemic proportions. Although these waves of infection were usually easy to treat—penicillin and other antibiotics seemed like magic bullets—some grew concerned.

Larry Kramer, the critically acclaimed gay novelist, playwright, and screenwriter, perhaps best known for the movie version of *Women in Love*, was one of the first to worry. He pleaded with his community to change its sexual behavior. "*Something* we are doing *is* ticking off the time bomb that is causing the breakdown of immunity in certain bodies," wrote Kramer in the *New York Native*, the city's gay weekly newspaper, in 1981. "While it is true that we don't know what it is specifically, isn't it better to be cautious until various suspected causes have been discounted, rather than be reckless?"

At first the answer was no, with some in the gay community choosing instead to shoot the messenger. He was lambasted as a fearmonger and a homophobe. "Read anything by Kramer closely," wrote Robert Chesley in a letter to the *Native*. "I think you'll find the subtext is always: the wages of gay sin are death."

But Kramer was not a lone voice crying in the wilderness. Joseph Sonnabend, in self-imposed exile from his native South Africa, had been a researcher and later director of Venereal Disease Control in New York City's Health Department before hanging out the shingle of private practice in Greenwich Village. Promiscuity was very prevalent among Sonnabend's clientele, and he soon began treating patients for a panoply of virulent infections. What he saw convinced him that danger lay ahead. He talked almost obsessively about the protective value of condoms. Initially his warnings went unheeded. Then the message grew more urgent.

The first published report gave no hint of an impending calamity, and the journal in which it appeared was not one to generate much public attention. On June 5, 1981, the Centers for Disease Control (CDC), the Atlanta-based federal public health agency charged with tracking

the spread of disease, described for the first time the unusual occurrence of *Pneumocystis carinii* pneumonia (PCP) in five gay men from
Los Angeles. Physicians who read *Morbidity and Mortality Weekly*
were startled; most had never encountered the rare pneumonia.

A month later, thousands got a more chilling portent of things to
come. On a July day that remains forever etched into so many memories, the *New York Times* ran an article that was headlined "Rare
Cancer Seen in 41 Homosexuals."

The cancer described in the *Times* was Kaposi's sarcoma, an obscure skin malignancy usually distinguished by reddish purple lesions
on the face, head, or mouth. Until the early 1980s, the disease was
hardly ever seen in people under the age of seventy and was rarely
fatal. Now, with "gay cancer" on the prowl, the untimely deaths of
a handful of healthy young men suddenly took on new meaning.

By the fall of 1981, physicians knew that PCP and Kaposi's sarcoma
were linked to something larger. A mysterious and deadly new syndrome, initially called Gay Related Immune Deficiency (GRID), was
afoot. Within a year, when similar virulent infections were observed
among drug users and hemophiliacs, the CDC gave the dreaded
disorder another name—Acquired Immune Deficiency Syndrome.

It became the toughest health challenge of the twentieth century. A
fatal illness was spiraling out of control. At first the political and
scientific establishment was unable to respond. The drug companies
sat quietly on the sidelines. Men and women with creativity, vision,
and the courage to shake up the status quo were in desperately short
supply. Risk-takers willing to use any means necessary to address an
unfolding public health disaster were few.

The absence of forceful direction at the highest levels of government power has been nothing less than criminal—and it remains so.
For the first four years of the epidemic, Ronald Reagan refused to
utter the word AIDS. Conservatives in charge at the White House
were so offended by gay lifestyles and sexual practices that a trickle
of AIDS cases was allowed to become a flood before any action was
taken. Racism and disdain for drug users, who are mainly poor and
often black and Hispanic, intensified the problem.

The government's response to AIDS is still characterized by an
almost total absence of aggressive leadership. George Bush's ascen-

sion to the presidency eight years into the epidemic has made little difference. Year after year, congressional investigators, prestigious commissions, and public health experts have examined the federal response to the epidemic and, year after year, they have said essentially the same thing: "No one is in charge. Put somebody in charge."

It has never happened. Instead, inside the circle of power, right-wing ideologues turned bigotry and hatred on hard-hit patients and their loved ones and their communities. They allowed a medical emergency to become tainted by a spirit of sanctimoniousness, then turned their backs as the disenfranchised began dying. To this day, there is still no single official or agency charged with developing a coherent national strategy on AIDS. That is a national disgrace.

The story of AIDS drug development has been focused partly on the cramped Rockville headquarters of the Food and Drug Administration (FDA), the Federal agency in charge of approving drugs for marketing, and also on the lush Bethesda campus of the National Institutes of Allergy and Infectious Diseases (NIAID), a few miles farther south, which took the lead role in testing promising AIDS drugs. Both the FDA and NIAID are institutions with noble goals. But their initial approach to AIDS was characterized by unconscionable foot-dragging.

For almost two years the FDA could not find a way to approve ganciclovir, a drug that prevented blindness, which everyone agreed worked safely and well. Meanwhile, NIAID so bungled its efforts to test pentamidine, used to prevent a lethal form of pneumonia, that activists and their physician allies had to seize the initiative and conduct tests on pentamidine themselves. It took the fury of the community to awaken these guardians of the public health to their errors and force change.

The response of the private sector was equally unimpressive. At first, AIDS generated little interest within the industry. It appeared to be a rare disease unworthy of the large investment necessary to bring a drug to market. In the absence of a tradition of corporate conscience, drug companies felt no obligation to address the needs of a public health catastrophe.

Then, in a story of greed and deceit, Burroughs Wellcome entered the picture. The pharmaceutical giant was lucky enough to hit the

jackpot with AZT, a drug developed by government scientists, which
the company happened to have sitting on its shelves. Here was a
therapy that allowed AIDS patients to eke out a few more years of
life—that is, if they could scrape together $10,000 a year to purchase
supplies of the drug. The company, after all, had to cash in while the
market was hot. It took Burroughs Wellcome's example of extraordinary profits to spark interest in AIDS from other drug companies. So
much for free enterprise.

From the beginning of the epidemic to the present, this combination of indifferent leadership, cumbersome bureaucracy, and corporate greed has had an impact almost as devastating as that of the
AIDS virus itself.

AIDS activism was a movement born of frustration and reared in
necessity. In the gay community, the epidemic initially spawned talk
of "beautiful death"; the notion of slipping peacefully from a world
of pain and sickness into one of eternal beauty was the rhetoric of the
early 1980s. In San Francisco, obituaries spoke in ethereal terms
about people journeying "to the other side," and "surrendering
Earth's sorrow." Treatment information, on the other hand, was
initially perceived as "quackery, false hope which interfered with the
process of accepting death," according to John James, who later
founded a newsletter about AIDS therapies.

That perspective began to shift as determination replaced passivity. The seeds of change were planted in the early, inertia-ridden days
of the epidemic, when Ronald Reagan refused to ask Congress to
allocate funds for AIDS. The gay community moved swiftly to fill the
vacuum in services, ministering to the sick and educating people to
the realities of an infectious and fatal new disease. One of the pioneers was Gay Men's Health Crisis, founded in 1981 in New York
City, largely to provide public health education, social support, and
counseling services. In its early years, resources were scarce and
internal struggles were often bitter, but today, more than a decade
after its start, GMHC is the largest and perhaps most widely known
community-based AIDS organization. On the West Coast, the San
Francisco AIDS Foundation was launched the same year, also to
provide direct services. It, too, remains in business.

Over the years, HIV-infected people in the gay middle class began refusing to be identified as AIDS "victims" or even "patients"; people living with AIDS, or PWAs, was the preferred description. Their worldwide changes in sexual behavior in response to the realities of the epidemic were among the swiftest in the history of public health. The self-help response to AIDS had an empowering effect, giving many a sense of their own possibilities and paving the way for more aggressive actions.

Among drug users, however, where rates of HIV infection were soaring, other health, economic, and social problems impeded their capacity to take control over their own lives. It was only those with the political acumen and wherewithal to seek treatments who first went outside the system to get unapproved drugs. Sophisticated smuggling networks and underground "drugstores" were established. While mainstream researchers struggled to find patients willing to enroll in poorly designed clinical trials, bootleggers were putting drugs into the hands of thousands.

Later, activists mobilized to push the bureaucracy to speed the research and approval of new therapies. The FDA, eviscerated by cutbacks during the Reagan years, was initially targeted as the source of the bottlenecks. Its laborious approval process sometimes allowed drugs to sit in limbo for months, even years before the data could be analyzed and judgment pronounced.

Often activists had the drug companies as their unlikely allies in their efforts to push the FDA as far as they could. Content at first to watch the FDA's regulatory authority wilt in the face of resource shortfalls, many in the private sector eventually became alarmed that the agency's impotence had begun to prevent their drugs from reaching the market. But the alliance between AIDS activists and pharmaceutical firms was always uneasy, and more than once, disputes over drug pricing shattered the ties.

Eventually AIDS activists became convinced that the obstacles at the FDA were only part of the problem; the dearth of promising drugs in the testing pipeline was equally disturbing. With that insight, they moved next to the National Institutes of Health, intent on targeting the drug development process at a much earlier stage. Here they used their bodies as leverage, telling researchers they would not participate in their studies unless they were given a decision-making voice in drug selection and trial design.

°   °   °

During the course of the struggle, AIDS has pushed some exceptional people to the frontlines.

Jim Eigo, a soft-spoken Lower East Side playwright, is one. The relationship he forged with Tony Fauci, a Brooklyn boy who had made good in the corridors of the Washington power elite and became head of NIAID, helped bridge the chasm between the activists and the scientific establishment.

Another unexpected bond was formed between Larry Kramer, the Angry Man of the AIDS movement, and Ellen Cooper, the scientist in charge of reviewing AIDS drugs for the FDA. At first, Kramer accused Cooper of "Nazi-like tactics." Later, as the two found common ground, rhetoric gave way to reconciliation and he called her a Joan of Arc.

Years before AIDS, Martin Delaney recovered from a serious illness by using an experimental drug. That experience, coupled with the agony of watching his lover struggle with AIDS, persuaded a man with no medical training to sponsor a secret trial of a dangerous Chinese drug called Compound Q. Martin Delaney, who almost became a Jesuit priest and easily might have been a millionaire businessman, chose instead to push the boundaries of law and ethics in the interest of human needs.

Another extraordinary player is activist Peter Staley, a Wall Street bond trader turned saboteur. For Staley, a self-described yuppie and once a Reaganite, it was simply a matter of life and death.

Also put in the spotlight was Mathilde Krim, a Swiss-born cancer researcher who launched the nation's largest private-sector foundation to fund AIDS research. Krim was driven into activism by old memories of another holocaust and the conviction that traditional scientific thinking often results in missed opportunities.

Together with many others, these people organized to fight against AIDS and in the process changed the American biomedical establishment in ways certain to transcend the epidemic. Their insistent demands led to an overhaul of mechanisms that put experimental therapies into patient hands. Activists also helped develop community-based research, a historic new approach to drug testing, and forced other big changes in how research is conducted.

So determined were the activists, and so sophisticated their knowledge of the bureaucratic and scientific realities of AIDS, that they were finally given a seat at the table of power. The seat remains rickety and the fight to change the system is far from over. But the empowerment of the AIDS patient community will surely last and will provide a model for others to follow.

In June 1990, Peter Staley addressed the International AIDS Conference in San Francisco. Some of his remarks had been prepared by the late Vito Russo, a film historian who was too ill with AIDS-related pneumonia to speak that day.

"AIDS is a test of who we are as a people," said Staley. "When future generations ask what we did in the war, we have to be able to tell them that we were out here fighting. And we have to leave a legacy to the generations of people who will come after us.

"Remember that someday the AIDS crisis will be over. And when that day has come and gone, there will be people alive on this earth— gay people and straight people, black people and white people, men and women—who will hear the story, that once there was a terrible disease, and that a brave group of people stood up and fought, and in some cases died, so that others might live and be free."

This is the story of those people and the war they are still fighting. It is also a tale of lost opportunities and deadly decisions and an account of how AIDS drug development has been enmeshed in a web of politics, profits, and business-as-usual bureaucracy. And finally, it is the story of the alliances that were forged to untangle it.

2

A NEW VIRUS

The Search for Magic Bullets

❖

I have a face in my mind for every AIDS-related
condition I can describe to you, and sometimes several
faces, every one the face of a friend.

—JIM EIGO,
AIDS activist

THE PERSONAL TRAGEDIES of a handful of public figures have helped
make AIDS real to millions of Americans. When movie star Rock
Hudson announced that he had AIDS, homosexuality suddenly
moved beyond the realm of an abstraction in the minds of those in the
mainstream. Likewise, basketball superstar Magic Johnson's courageous announcement in November 1991 that he had been infected
with the virus that causes AIDS, probably through one of his numerous heterosexual encounters, brought the truth about the epidemic
chillingly close to home.

By communicating the message that no one was invulnerable to
AIDS, Rock Hudson and Magic Johnson sought to foster greater
compassion. The tragic story of a young Florida woman named Kimberly Bergalis, by contrast, fueled a terrible divisiveness in the public
discourse.

The circumstances surrounding Bergalis's illness were unusual: she was the first person believed to be infected by her dentist, and this is considered to be an extremely rare mode of transmission. Unfortunately, Bergalis chose to use the public attention her story attracted to call for mandatory testing of all health-care workers to determine whether they carried the AIDS virus. Although her call was echoed by Jesse Helms and other conservative forces in Congress, mandatory testing is widely believed to be costly, ineffective, and punitive— exactly the wrong societal response to the devastation of AIDS. More significantly, Bergalis's us-against-them attitude sought to divide people with AIDS into two camps—those who had done "something wrong" to bring the disease upon themselves, and the innocent victims of forces they were powerless to control. Bergalis apparently believed that true compassion was deserved only by innocents such as herself.

Despite her blind-sided politics, Bergalis's poignant account of suffering reflected the agony of hundreds of thousands dead or dying from AIDS. In a letter released to the press as she lingered near death, Bergalis wrote:

> When I was diagnosed with AIDS in December of '89, I was only twenty-one years old. It was the shock of my life and my family's as well. I have lived to see my hair fall out, my body lose over forty pounds, blisters on my sides. I've lived to go through nausea and vomiting, continual night sweats, chronic fevers of 103–104 that don't go away anymore. I have cramping and diarrhea. I now have convulsions and forgetfulness. I have endured trips twice a week to Miami for three months only to receive painful IV injections. I've had blood transfusions. I've had bone marrow biopsy. I cried my heart out from the pain of the biopsy.
>
> I lived through the fear of whether or not my liver has been completely destroyed by ddI and other drugs. It may very well be. I lived to see white fungus grow all over the inside of my mouth, the back of my throat, my gums, and now my lips. It looks like white fur and it gives you atrocious breath. Isn't that nice? I have tiny blisters on my lips. It may be the first stages of herpes. . . .
>
> Have you ever awakened in the middle of the night soaking wet from a night sweat—only to have it happen again an hour later? Can you imagine what it's like to realize you're losing weight in your fingers and that your body may be using its muscles to try to survive? Or do you

know what it's like to look at yourself in a full-length mirror before you shower—and you only see a skeleton? Do you know what I did? I slid to the floor and I cried. Now I shower with a blanket over the mirror. . . .

I'm dying. . . .

The few well-publicized tragedies left many Americans wondering why effective AIDS treatments were so hard to find. It will take a historian's perspective to determine which obstacles reflected the complexities of science and which were functions of an unresponsive bureaucracy and corporate greed; both clearly played a role. But aggressive drug research could not even begin until the virus that caused AIDS had been identified and scientific knowledge about the course of the disease was sharpened.

HIV: DISCOVERY AND CONTROVERSY

The first breakthrough in AIDS research came in May 1983 when scientists isolated a new virus while treating Frédéric Brugière, a Parisian fashion designer who had fallen ill. The new virus was soon dubbed BRU, in the designer's honor, and twelve French scientists, mainly from the Pasteur Institute in Paris, described it in a scientific journal.

But the French team's discovery was largely ignored, partly because there was no sure proof that their viral isolate was directly linked to AIDS. Besides, media and scientific attention was focused across the Atlantic, where Robert Gallo, chief of the Tumor Cell Biology lab at the National Cancer Institute, was hard at work. Gallo thought AIDS was somehow related to HTLV, the leukemia virus discovered in his lab a few years earlier. Eventually, Gallo isolated a virus from AIDS patients that he labeled HTLV-IIIB.

The French and the Americans studied their respective viruses intensively. Each made significant strides toward establishing them as the cause of AIDS. The first hint that something unusual had occurred came when the detailed genetic sequences of both viruses were published. Virologists were astonished at the similarities of their structure. Given that viruses are constantly mutating, the probability was almost nil that two laboratories thousands of miles apart would isolate identical viral strains.

Because the French and the Americans had earlier exchanged isolates of BRU and HTLV-IIIB, suspicions were quickly aroused. A rumor in scientific circles was that Gallo had stolen the French virus, then claimed to have isolated it himself.

Gallo maintained that BRU and HTLV-IIIB were actually different viral strains, despite their remarkable similarities. In 1984, nearly a year after the French discovery, Margaret Heckler, then Secretary of Health and Human Services, declared Gallo the true discoverer of the virus.

The French were inflamed, especially after the lucrative patent for an antibody test kit—a market now worth more than $100 million a year in the United States alone—was awarded to the U.S. government. Cries of scientific fraud burst into the open. So heated was the debate that two heads of state had to intervene. In 1987, President Ronald Reagan and Jacques Chirac, the prime minister of France, inked a historic agreement that gave equal credit to the Americans and the French for discovering the virus. By then an international committee, given the job of naming the virus, had designated it human immunodeficiency virus, or HIV. The settlement called for royalties from the HIV antibody test kit to be split on a fifty-fifty basis between the two nations.

But the doubters were not silenced. In a 50,000-word *Chicago Tribune* pull-out supplement in November 1989, John Crewdson, a Pulitzer Prize–winning investigative reporter, concluded that either laboratory contamination had allowed Gallo to mistake the French sample for his own viral isolate, or that Gallo had knowingly swiped the French virus and called it his own. Crewdson wrote: "Officially the dispute has been settled forever. In reality, the scientific world has been left with more questions than answers about who really discovered the cause of AIDS, and when and where and how. . . .

"What happened in Robert Gallo's lab during the winter of 1983–84 is a mystery that may never be entirely solved. But the evidence is compelling that it was either an accident or a theft."

Crewdson was wrong; the dispute was not settled forever. His article launched a new round of government inquiries.

In May 1991, another theory was advanced. Gallo and Luc Montagnier, one of the Pasteur Institute researchers, said that BRU and HTLV-IIIB had each been accidentally contaminated by a third virus, known as HIV-LAI, taken from the body of a French patient. That virus is known to grow well in laboratory cultures, and so it was not unusual that it had contaminated both viruses. That consensus seemed likely at last to still the voices of doubt and bring an end to seven years of innuendo and strife.

Despite the brouhaha over its discovery, most scientists have accepted HIV as the cause of AIDS. A handful of dissenters, however, still argue that the disease is not the work of a single virus but of a combination of interrelated factors. Joe Sonnabend, for example, has speculated that AIDS develops after a barrage of commonplace sexually transmitted diseases has so assaulted the immune system that the body cannot fight back.

Michael Callen credits Sonnabend's theory with keeping him alive. Callen, a long-term AIDS survivor and activist, estimates that by the time of his diagnosis in 1982, he'd had more than 3,000 sexual partners and shared countless venereal diseases with them. "Believing that a killer virus was responsible for my illness made my survival prospects seem grim and sapped my willingness to put up a fight," wrote Callen in *Surviving AIDS*, in which he profiles people who defy the medical odds to live many years with AIDS. By contrast, he said that Sonnabend's theory bolstered him with a sense of control, providing "a life raft that kept me afloat in a sea of doom and gloom."

Other theories about the cause of AIDS continue to be advanced. Peter Duesberg, a respected molecular biologist in California, echoed Sonnabend's view that, given enough time and enough battering, the human immune system eventually breaks down. Another important voice of dissent was, ironically, that of Luc Montagnier, who startled the scientific community in 1990 by disputing the prevailing consensus. Montagnier speculated that a mycoplasma, a minute microorganism believed to be a primitive bacteria, may have to be present, together with HIV, for AIDS to develop.

Despite such nagging doubts, scientific and pharmaceutical research has proceeded on the widely held assumption that HIV is the cause of AIDS.

* * *

HIV is probably the most thoroughly analyzed virus in the history of medicine. Its molecular and genetic structure have been closely scrutinized, its life cycle assiduously studied to determine where and when it is most susceptible to chemical weaponry.

Like other viruses, HIV can reproduce only by hijacking the biochemical machinery of the host cell. Typically, genetic information passes either from one DNA strand to another (DNA being the nucleic acid in the nucleus of human cells that carries all the body's genetic information) or from DNA to RNA (the nucleic acid that directs protein synthesis).

HIV, however, is a retrovirus, an extraordinary class of viruses that converts its genetic information in a backward flow from RNA to DNA. This trick is accomplished through a biologically unique enzyme called reverse transcriptase, which acts after HIV has penetrated the T cells. The unusual enzyme was discovered by two scientists, Howard Temin and David Baltimore, who won a Nobel Prize for their work in 1975. Once reverse transcriptase causes a DNA copy of the viral RNA to be made, the genetic code can be incorporated into the host cells. Eventually, after a period of latency that can last many years, the virus begins to replicate and infect other cells. At least two genes—known as Tat and Rev—and possibly others, must be present to trigger viral activity.

HIV wreaks its damage by targeting the cells of the immune system. Like a key and a lock, a virus and a host cell must fit together for the virus to slip inside. The key is the outer protein coating of HIV, and the lock is the CD4 protein. The CD4 protein is particularly profuse on the helper T lymphocytes, a subset of white blood cells manufactured in the bone marrow and programmed to counter microbes and other tiny invaders. HIV also goes after macrophages, which constitute another crucial component of the body's early-warning system.

Because HIV destroys CD4 cells, a CD4 count is a critical barometer of immune system function. Healthy adults typically have CD4 counts that range from 800 to 2,200. The danger zone for HIV-infected people, when disease is likely to develop, begins when counts drop to 500 and intensifies as the count plummets below 200.

◦   ◦   ◦

As the term is defined by the Centers for Disease Control, AIDS actually represents only one end of a long spectrum of HIV-related illnesses. Although this official definition is used to count incidence of disease and is the basis for Medicaid eligibility, Social Security disability, and other government benefits, many infected patients die without ever being formally diagnosed with AIDS. In 1991 the CDC proposed a revision of the definition of AIDS to include any HIV-infected person with a count of 200 or fewer CD4 cells. When the new definition is implemented, it will expand the number of AIDS diagnoses, although many drug users, who lack access to medical care and are often unaware of their CD4 cell counts, will surely die without becoming AIDS statistics.

It is impossible to predict just when someone infected by HIV will develop signs of illness—often it takes many years—but the incubation period is not a time of tranquility. "Being HIV positive and asymptomatic is like living with a constant, low-level crisis," said one patient. "It's a time bomb that may or may not go off at any point."

Once the time bomb explodes, there is almost no part of the human body that is not vulnerable to a cancer or an infection somehow linked to HIV. The lungs, heart, brain, kidneys, and gastrointestinal system can all be sites of disease. Infections also develop in the mouth, skin, eyes, nose, joints, muscles, glands, and elsewhere.

The course of the disease is unpredictable. For months or even years, between bouts of illness, a patient can be relatively free of symptoms. At other times the body is battered by simultaneous and often virulent diseases—known as opportunistic infections—as viruses, bacteria, fungi, and parasites take advantage of the body's weakened capacity to defend itself. Some of these are life-threatening, others excruciatingly painful. Many of these diseases are easily treatable if a patient is otherwise healthy, yet can kill someone with HIV. Some, like tuberculosis, had been steadily declining before AIDS but have now reached epidemic proportions again.

Pinning down just how long the period is from point of infection until a patient develops the range of symptoms that have been defined as AIDS is extremely difficult because there's seldom a way to know with certainty when someone was first infected. On the basis of a handful of studies, researchers estimate the wait typically ranges from eight to eleven years. What's more certain is that once symptoms appear, death usually follows within a few years.

THE SEARCH FOR DRUGS

The focus of current AIDS research falls into two broad categories: the search for antiviral drugs that are targeted directly at HIV, and the search for drugs designed to treat the multitude of accompanying infections. A third group of drugs, known as immune enhancers or immunoregulators, boost the body's defense system but also can stimulate viral replication, which has hampered productive research.

Because AIDS manifests itself in so many different ways, no single drug is likely ever to cure the disease. Most scientists believe the key to treating AIDS, like the key to treating cancer, will be the effective use of multiple therapies to keep HIV in check and stave off opportunistic infections or treat those that occur. The tools to do the job are still woefully inadequate.

Between 1987 and 1991 the National Cancer Institute tested 40,000 chemical compounds at facilities in Frederick, Maryland, and Birmingham, Alabama, to see if any could disable the AIDS virus. Despite the odds against finding a breakthrough drug, researchers continue to screen for compounds that can inhibit HIV at each step in the infection process: when it binds to the CD4 molecule; when it penetrates the helper T cell; when it transcribes its genetic code inside; and when it replicates. A more promising direction for future research is targeted drug development—that is, designing an effective drug based on the known biological structure of HIV.

Unfortunately, the complexity of the virus makes both screening and targeted drug development extraordinarily difficult. To be effective, an antiviral drug would most likely have to be administered early in the course of HIV infection, before the immune system has been too thoroughly impaired. Or methods to restore damaged immune function would have to be developed, an avenue of research that is not far advanced. And even if an effective drug were found, HIV's devilishly clever capacity to mutate, and thus to evade pharmaceutical attack, might soon render it worthless.

* * *

By 1992 the most widely used antiviral drugs were nucleoside analogues, a family of synthetic compounds that inhibit the reverse transcriptase enzyme, preventing the virus from copying its genetic information into newly infected cells. These drugs—including AZT
(azidothymidine), ddI (dideoxyinosine), and ddC (dideoxycytidine)—
cannot repair already damaged cells or prevent all opportunistic infections, but they do extend life.

On March 17, 1987, AZT became the first anti-HIV therapy to be
licensed by the FDA. For more than four years that drug, sold by
Burroughs Wellcome, was the only approved treatment, and its story
highlights much that is both right and wrong about AIDS drug research.

Although it can prolong life, AZT has proven toxic to bone marrow,
often causing anemia severe enough to necessitate blood transfusions
and forcing patients off the drug. Severe headache, nausea, insomnia,
and muscle pain are also common side effects, and AZT-resistant
strains of HIV are likely to limit the drug's value. These drawbacks
kept scientists focused on antiviral alternatives, but years dragged by
before there was an addition to the therapeutic arsenal.

Finally, on October 9, 1991, after an intensive committment of
resources, the FDA approved Bristol-Myers's application to market
ddI. The agency was also moving aggressively to review Hoffman–La
Roche's ddC application, which was being submitted in stages to
speed up the process. DdI and ddC both increase CD4 cell counts but
are also associated with peripheral neuropathy, a tingling, numbing,
and burning of the extremities, especially the feet. Worse, ddI can
cause pancreatitis, an acute inflammation of the pancreas, which can
be lethal. Still, ddI has been one of the rare success stories in AIDS
drug development. Its approval demonstrated that patients can be
given experimental therapies without jeopardizing good science and
that philosophical changes at the FDA were finally being translated
into tangible regulatory achievements.

Four other compounds that inhibit the reverse transcriptase enzyme initially generated tremendous excitement within the patient
community. Foscarnet, approved to treat cytomegalovirus retinitis on
September 27, 1991, continued to look promising against HIV but the
other three drugs—suramin, HPA-23, and ribavirin—were eventu-

ally discredited. Nonetheless, each one provoked a significant response within the patient community and for that reason earned a spot in AIDS history.

Another promising avenue of antiviral research involves blocking the binding of HIV to the CD4 protein.

One drug, long stalled in the testing pipeline, is Peptide T, which occupies the cellular site where the virus would otherwise attach itself. Developed in 1986 by Candace Pert and other government scientists, Peptide T is a short chain of amino acids that was synthesized in the laboratory to match part of the protein sequences of HIV itself. Despite Pert's passionate commitment to the drug, she was unable to push it into a major trial for four years; charges were made that the delay was caused by professional rivalries or the vested financial interests of certain researchers.

Although they have not held up to scientific scrutiny, dextran sulfate and AL-721 both bolstered the AIDS underground, earning them a notoriety that transcends their therapeutic value. In the laboratory, dextran sulfate, a long chain of sugar molecules, attaches itself to a host cell and confers negative charges to repel HIV. It may also inhibit production of the reverse transcriptase enzyme. But researchers have been unable to duplicate those results in human trials because the drug is not well absorbed in the bloodstream. AL-721's clinical effectiveness is also in doubt. The drug, composed entirely of substances found in egg yolk, increases the fluidity of proteins on the membrane of the T cells, preventing the virus from attaching itself to the altered membrane.

The first major targeted AIDS drug development effort used the tools of biotechnology to create a synthetic CD4 molecule. The recombinant molecule uses its own key to open the lock of the CD4 molecule on the T cell, blocking HIV from doing so instead. Unfortunately, clinical trial results with the synthetic molecule were disappointing and early enthusiasm has waned.

Alpha interferon, now licensed for use in AIDS patients with Kaposi's sarcoma, looks more promising and further studies are under way. A big plus for interferon, a human protein that can now be genetically engineered, is its range of activity; along with its action against KS lesions, it inhibits HIV's last stage of viral reproduction.

Another controversial antiviral drug is GLQ-223, a protein toxin from the root of the Chinese cucumber plant, which gained widespread notoriety when patient activists discarded many of the norms of scientific practice to test it. Popularly known as Compound Q, it is still being studied to determine whether it can dispatch the reservoirs of virus stored in the macrophages—a key component of the immune system's early-warning line of defense—without damaging healthy cells.

Despite the lengthy list of antivirals under study, the tale of AIDS drug development is in a sense just beginning. Only now, as the world moves into the second decade of the epidemic, are we truly armed with both the biomedical knowledge and a flexible enough research and approval system to make real headway.

A cure for AIDS is unlikely anytime soon. The focus of treatment and research now is to achieve a delicate balance among several antiviral therapies. It is hoped that the right combination of drugs will reduce cumulative toxicities and lengthen the period during which treatment is effective.

At the same time, opportunistic infections will need to be treated more aggressively. Because each one has to be handled individually—and most infections typically assault only a fraction of the HIV-infected population—it has generally been hard to entice drug companies or scientists into this research.

Still, some progress has been made. People with AIDS now live years longer than they did in the early 1980s. They live more comfortably as well, with therapies that improve quality of life and extend the years of relatively good health. The time from infection to the onset of symptoms has been lengthened by the early use of drugs, and certain killer infections have been brought under control. Scientists continue to hope that AIDS will someday be transformed from an almost inevitably fatal disease to a survivable chronic illness.

The other great hope is for a vaccine. Jonas Salk, credited with inventing the polio vaccine, has reemerged from relative obscurity to join this quest, but numerous scientific challenges block the way. Since a vaccine is likely to use some component of the AIDS virus, the first challenge is to avoid infecting healthy people. Even getting vaccine trials off the ground has been tough; volunteers willing to be injected with any form of HIV are, not surprisingly, few in number. An alternative approach is to inject already infected people with a vaccine in hopes of boosting their immune systems. But scientists still don't know enough about stimulating effective antibodies, nor do they know which HIV proteins to use in the vaccine.

Politics and profits are as likely as science to impede the development of a vaccine. Many drug companies are reluctant to invest in research that might backfire dramatically and infect healthy people or hasten the deaths of HIV-infected ones. The federal government will likely have to indemnify industry against liability before a vaccine is ever marketed.

Still, the potential worldwide market for an effective vaccine is enormous. Few drugs hold the profit potential of a vaccine that could guarantee protection against the deadly AIDS virus. Although small biotechnology firms have done most of the preliminary research, the big pharmaceutical companies are not likely to linger long on the sidelines.

Not with all that money to be made. That hasn't been the pattern of AIDS drug development.

3

THE FDA AND THE PUBLIC INTEREST

You just got bad blood and we is trying to help you.

—Nurse to Alabama
sharecropper in
*Bad Blood: The Tuskegee
Syphilis Experiment,* by
James H. Jones

THE AMERICAN APPROACH to regulating and approving new drugs has a well-deserved reputation as rigorous, probably the most rigorous in the world. The Food and Drug Administration is in charge. But its process has historically been slow and cumbersome, more adept at keeping bad drugs off the market than at speeding up access to good ones. Rock Hudson's desperate dash to Paris to obtain HPA-23 gave the public an early inkling of a complex problem.

HPA-23—its scientific name is antimoniotungstate—is an antiviral drug developed in the early 1970s that seemed to interfere with the chemical process involved in HIV replication. Michael Gottlieb, Hudson's physician, had read about HPA-23, which was being tested at the Pasteur Institute, and tried to interest American drug companies in looking into it further. But he quickly learned that in the mid-1980s the drug industry was still not interested in AIDS research.

Rock Hudson despaired of finding a domestic source of HPA-23 and chartered a jet across the Atlantic in pursuit of a cure.

The value of HPA-23 was never proven, but Hudson's odyssey alerted Americans that certain drugs could sometimes be secured overseas many years before they maneuvered through the convoluted drug testing and approval process at home.

Contrary to popular assumption, the FDA does not actually conduct human research, although it frequently advises drug companies on trial design. Once testing is complete and an application is submitted, the FDA takes an average of thirty months to reach an approval decision on the new drug.

A commitment to rigorous science is one reason so much time elapses. A shortage of resources also has a lot to do with it. The FDA does not have the budget or the personnel to do its job properly. Every commission and congressional investigation—and there have been scores of them in the past decade—has reached essentially that same conclusion. The annual AIDS research budget of the National Institutes of Health soared from $5.5 million in 1982 to $807 million in 1991, a stunning increase of more than 14,000 percent. During roughly the same time, the FDA's budget stayed almost flat in constant dollars.

Meanwhile, Congress loaded the agency with new responsibilities, passing thirty-two laws that affect the FDA during the past decade. Twelve of those laws were passed in 1990 alone. At the same time the agency has been swamped by obligations to respond to overseers. By one count, the FDA was the subject of eighty-four congressional hearings and fifty-nine federal studies between 1985 and 1990. An explosion in private-sector pharmaceutical research further burdened the FDA, which had to review more drugs than ever before; it approved a record 792 drugs in 1988. Although that figure fell to 465 the following year and to 229 in 1990, a tidal wave of new product applications—especially in the swiftly evolving field of biotechnology—was expected. The agency wasn't even close to having the capacity to meet the demand.

Some new employees were finally brought on board in the late 1980s to handle the burgeoning responsibilities imposed by AIDS, but the agency remained grossly understaffed and underfunded. In 1991 the agency had a $682-million budget and 8,400 full-time employees. The federal General Accounting Office has said the FDA now needs to increase its staff by 2,000 people to do its mandated job appropriately. With an eye to the future, the FDA's own management team predicts that by 1997 a work force of 17,000 people and a budget of $2 billion will be required to do its job effectively.

Workspace at the FDA is woefully inadequate. Employees are spread among thirty-two different buildings at eleven different sites in the Washington area, and the agency's offices and laboratory facilities are overcrowded, outdated, unsafe, and poorly maintained. Scientific equipment is obsolete and technologically inadequate. Just how dire the situation was brought vividly home to Admiral James D. Watkins, chairman of the Presidential Commission on the HIV Epidemic, which was appointed by Ronald Reagan in 1987 to assess the public health dimensions of AIDS and to examine its medical, legal, ethical, social, and economic impact. When Watkins toured FDA facilities, scientists pulled him into back rooms to plead privately for more staff, more equipment, and more resources. Watkins commented afterward that the place looked like a "Third World research institute."

The consensus was clear: more money was desperately needed. Even pharmaceutical executives, who had traditionally been hostile toward FDA mandates, were disturbed enough by lengthy delays and regulatory inconsistencies to call for heightened funding levels. But new resources were not likely to be forthcoming. At least not from the debt-laden Bush Administration.

Until World War II, medical research was little more than a cottage industry. Local physicians typically experimented on themselves, on family members, or on neighbors. If an unapproved treatment turned out to be effective, the research subjects were the direct beneficiaries.

That began to change during the war. For the first time, large numbers of basically healthy subjects were enlisted in experiments designed to find treatments for others. Most of the participants came from jails, mental hospitals, and other institutions charged with caring for society's most vulnerable members. Participation in medical experiments became more burden than benefit, especially for disenfranchised populations. Egregious tales of abuse were common.

Under the federal Office of Scientific Research and Development, created by President Franklin D. Roosevelt in 1941, some $25 million in medical research contracts were let during the war years. Most of the funds went to find antidotes to dysentery, influenza, venereal diseases, and malaria, which were disabling many American soldiers overseas and threatening the war efforts. "Asylum wards where dysentery was endemic were substituted as the setting of research, and no one objected to experiments on impaired inmates. In fact, researchers with links to custodial institutions had an edge in securing grants," wrote David Rothman, a medical historian at Columbia University. Typical was Contract 120, carried out at the New Jersey State Colony for the Feeble-Minded, where retarded residents were used to test treatments for dysentery.

A similarly outrageous experiment was conducted by University of Chicago researchers, who established a sixty-bed unit at Mantero Illinois State Hospital, where they deliberately infected psychotic patients with malaria through blood transfusions. These patients were then given anti-malarial remedies, and the results studied. In an Illinois state penitentiary, 500 prisoners were "volunteered" to participate in malaria research. In Pennsylvania, residents of a state facility for the retarded and young offenders at a nearby correctional center were given influenza shots, then injected with a flu virus to test the vaccine's effectiveness.

In the prevailing wartime mood—personal sacrifices were expected and a sense of urgency prevailed—few paused to question the ethics of such research. The operative notion was that in the fight for democracy, everyone had a role to play. Or, as Rothman wrote, "Some people were ordered to face bullets and storm a hill; others were told to take an injection and test a vaccine." When it came to testing prisoners, "the public response was not to ask whether prisoners were able to give voluntary consent but to congratulate 'these one-time enemies to society' for demonstrating 'to the fullest extent possible just how completely this is everybody's war.'"

Slowly, public attitudes toward the ethics of research began to shift. When the Nazis' mutilating, inhuman experiments were revealed, attention became focused on the urgent need to protect a subject's welfare. The Nuremberg Code, set forth in 1949, defined the structure of an ethical experiment. Under the code, the humanitarian importance of an experiment was required to outweigh its risks, the research had to be designed so that it was likely to yield fruitful results, and research subjects had to be afforded reasonable protection from injury. Above all, participants had to be able to give competent, voluntary, and informed consent and be allowed to quit the trial at any time.

Despite the Nuremberg Code, the pattern of human experimentation established in this country during World War II was slow to change. In a famous article published in 1966, Henry Beecher, a Harvard University anesthesiologist, described twenty-two research projects that had endangered participants. Beecher's article went far in fostering public revulsion toward unethical experiments, particularly since his examples came from mainstream research sponsored by leading medical schools, university hospitals, and governmental agencies, including the National Institutes of Health, the Veterans Administration, and the army, navy, and air force. Subjects included soldiers in the armed forces, hospitalized charity patients, mentally retarded children, the terminally ill, the elderly, and chronic alcoholics. Many of the participants suffered grave and permanent damage from their involvement in medical experiments, yet had been told little about possible risks. Some did not even know they were part of a study.

A common practice described by Beecher was the withholding of treatment known to be effective to allow scientists to study the course of a disease; in one experiment, servicemen were denied penicillin to heighten the odds that they would develop rheumatic fever after a respiratory infection. In other flagrant abuses, patients were deliberately given toxic drugs, asked to swallow ammonia, injected with live cancer cells, exposed to excess levels of X rays, and pierced through the heart with a needle—all in the name of advancing science.

The Tuskegee syphilis study exposed by Jean Heller of the Associated Press in 1972 was a further shocker. Heller uncovered a study sponsored by the United States government in which hundreds of black men in Macon County, Alabama, were diagnosed with syphilis—then left untreated for forty years so that researchers could monitor the course of their disease. The progression of syphilis had already been established in studies published in Europe, but scientists weren't convinced those findings could be generalized to nonwhites. Since the virulent venereal disease leads to blindness, insanity, and death in its late stages, the Tuskegee experiment was nothing less than government-sanctioned abuse.

Such horror stories eventually led to a loud cry for reform. By 1974, Congress had created the National Commission for the Protection of Human Subjects of Biomedical and Behavioral Research. Four years later the commission issued the Belmont Report, which defined the ethical principles that became the foundation for drug research. The report made a special point of warning researchers not to abuse vulnerable populations, including poor people, minorities, and the institutionalized. Traditionally these groups were systematically selected for medical experiments because they had been easy to find, easy to manipulate, or incapable of saying no.

Drug research was generally required to fit within the Belmont framework—until AIDS shook the whole system to its foundation.

The sordid roots of medical research and regulation have parallels in the evolution of the drug approval process. The system of testing drugs and okaying them for marketing also developed in response to negligence that was sometimes deliberate, other times merely careless.

Until the early part of the twentieth century, virtually no national regulations governed the sale of drugs. Although some state and local governments enforced their own laws, drugs were generally advertised directly to the public and could be purchased without a prescription. Much of what was available was simply worthless; other products were toxic. Medicines containing opium, morphine, heroin, and cocaine were peddled openly to consumers.

The federal laws passed since the 1900s, almost always in response to catastrophe, gradually created the FDA's regulatory framework that today has a few staunch defenders, more inflamed critics, and a great many advocates of at least modest reform.

The Pure Food and Drugs Act, the first major piece of national legislation in this field, forbade manufacturers from making unsubstantiated claims on medicine labels. But the 1906 statute was almost toothless. The burden of proof to show that a drug was labeled fraudulently rested with the government, and the law did not "require pre-market approval, pre-market testing, pre-market notification, or indeed pre-market anything," according to Peter Barton

Hutt, formerly chief counsel to the FDA. "A drug manufacturer under the 1906 act did not even have to inform the Food and Drug Administration [actually known as the Bureau of Chemistry at the time and lodged in the Department of Agriculture] that it was in business."

In 1927 the Bureau of Chemistry was reorganized as the Food, Drug and Insecticide Administration, which in turn became the Food and Drug Administration four years later. There were few drug regulations on the books. During the Depression, when medical quackery blossomed into a source of income for some of the nation's destitute, and scandal broke upon wave of scandal, public support finally began to build for more stringent controls on drugs. With backing from several national women's organizations, the FDA lobbied for tougher legislation, presenting an investigating Senate committee with a set of horror stories. One concerned a Pittsburgh steel magnate who died after drinking a poisoned bottle of radium water labeled in accordance with then-current law.

For five years new legislation was introduced into Congress, but for five years the bills were shot down, thanks mostly to strenuous protests from pharmaceutical companies.

Then, in 1937, tragedy struck. Sulfa "wonder drugs" had come into widespread use, and Massengill, a Tennessee-based manufacturer, was looking for a leg up in the market. Somewhere in the company's executive suites it was decided that patients, especially children, preferred to take medication in liquid form. Chemists got busy looking for a solvent that would dissolve the active drug in their sulfa product, and eventually settled on diethylene glycol, which is normally used in radiator antifreeze. After a bit of artificial color and raspberry flavoring were added, the product appeared on drugstore shelves under the name Elixir Sulfanilamide. In short order, more than 100 people had died in agony from kidney failure linked directly to the poisonous solvent.

A subsequent investigation revealed that no product safety tests had ever been run on the product. It wasn't even clear that the chemists had consulted standard textbooks to learn more about diethylene glycol. Although the company's chief chemist committed suicide soon after the Elixir Sulfanilamide scandal, Massengill accepted no formal culpability. After all, the 1906 act didn't require safety checks.

The ensuing public outcry forced the passage of the Food, Drug and Cosmetic Act the following year, at last making it illegal to market a drug until it had been proven safe. The act, which provides the framework for FDA operations to this day, also barred manufacturers from making false claims for their drugs and required that labels contain adequate warnings and appropriate directions for use.

The legislation coincided with an explosive growth in the field of medicine. By the mid-1940s, penicillin and other antibiotics had been introduced, setting the stage for the golden era of drug development. Under the Food, Drug and Cosmetic Act, the new regulations for testing promising pharmaceuticals were simple; the FDA required merely that investigational drugs be appropriately labeled and used by expert scientists with adequate facilities who swore to use the drugs only for experimental purposes. In order to sell their drugs to the public, pharmaceutical companies had only to prove they were safe. There was no requirement that they also be effective. That made it easy to bring hundreds of new drugs to the market every year.

The FDA was a lean agency in the years following the enactment of the Food, Drug and Cosmetic Act. Just one physician monitored all investigational new drugs and approved all new drug applications. The agency typically spent about seven months reviewing data on a new product before allowing it to be sold. In 1955 the FDA's budget stood at $5.2 million. By 1960, with an $11-million budget, six full-time and four part-time physicians, the FDA was still far from a bloated bureaucracy.

The need for a tougher regulatory agency became apparent as abuses by pharmaceutical manufacturers began to surface. Senator Estes Kefauver, chair of the Subcommittee on Antitrust and Monopoly, waged a lonely battle to clamp down on the drug industry. Beginning in December 1959, his subcommittee held hearings that dragged on for twenty-six months and eventually filled 12,885 pages of government records.

Kefauver focused first on industry violations of the public trust. Witnesses from academia, government, and industry exposed shocking stories about price gouging, stock manipulation, advertising fraud, collusion with the FDA, and widespread deception. Claiming corporate profits were outrageous, Kefauver lobbied hard for government control over drug prices. As exposé built upon exposé, the senator broadened his focus and began pushing for proof that a drug worked before it could be given the FDA stamp of approval. But his proposed amendments to the Food, Drug and Cosmetic Act, designed to bolster the FDA's regulatory authority, did not generate much interest at first. Not in the pro-business climate prevailing during the Eisenhower Administration.

Then came thalidomide. The drug was marketed as a sedative in Europe and Canada in the late 1950s. Although it was never approved in the United States, more than 1,000 doctors managed to get hold of it. An estimated 20,000 Americans—including 624 who were pregnant and more than 3,000 other women of childbearing age— were actually given the drug, according to congressional reports. It was not long before thalidomide's tragic side effect became obvious— it caused terrible deformities in newborns. Dramatic news reports and disturbing photographs from Europe brought public attention to the thalidomide tragedy and provoked cries of outrage here.

Capitalizing on the spotlight focused on the drug industry, Kefauver pushed hard for his legislative initiatives. Some dissented. The amendments were called an encroachment by government into the traditional domain of medicine. The American Medical Association claimed that demanding proof of effectiveness before making a drug available for sale violated a patient's freedom to choose. But it was an election year, and regulation was finally in vogue. President John Kennedy endorsed the Kefauver Amendments in a public address to the nation, and Congress passed them without a single dissenting vote. On October 10, 1962, they were signed into law.

For the first time in American history, the federal government demanded proof not only that a drug was safe but that it worked. And for the next twenty-five years the Kefauver Amendments stood unchallenged.

CHALLENGING RESTRICTIONS ON EXPERIMENTAL DRUGS

Under the darkening cloud of AIDS, many people again began to oppose the FDA's efficacy requirements. So long as a drug is safe, they said, it should be made available to all who want it. Even if it is worthless.

"It is as if I am in a disabled airplane, speeding downward out of control," said one patient in a journal article. "I see a parachute hanging on the cabin wall, one small moment of hope. I try to strap it on when a government employee reaches out and tears it off my back, admonishing, 'You can't use that. It doesn't have a Federal Aviation Administration inspection sticker on it. We don't know if it will work.'"

In discussions about expanding access to unproven drugs, two extreme positions were staked out. At one end were those who argued that even in the face of AIDS, the FDA should never distribute a drug until it has passed the rigorous, three-phase testing process that takes many years to complete. Distributing drugs any earlier, claimed this faction, subjects patients to unacceptable risks and jeopardizes the time-honored system of testing drugs. But as the AIDS epidemic gathered force, this became a distinctly minority point of view.

Then there were political ideologues who essentially called for the dismantling of the FDA. Sam Kazman, chief counsel for the Competitive Enterprise Institute, a conservative think tank, was one of those at the other end of the spectrum. In a *Washington Post* op-ed piece, Kazman urged the FDA to announce "that it will no longer stand between AIDS sufferers and the medicines they seek; that people with AIDS are free to obtain what they can from doctors, drug companies, researchers and so forth."

Kazman proposed that the FDA relinquish all authority to keep drugs off the market; instead, he suggested the agency certify drugs that had met its safety and effectiveness standards and make others available with a warning about their unapproved status. "Those who wished to rely on the FDA's judgment could continue to do so. The rest of us could knowingly and contractually assume the risks of unconventional therapies," Kazman wrote.

Most academics, policymakers, patient advocates, and medical ethicists sought a middle ground—a place where the public was protected from unsafe or worthless drugs while at least some people with AIDS could get access to promising but unproven treatments. This had historically been the FDA's position with cancer and there was pressure to apply the policy more broadly.

*   *   *

One staunch believer in a patient's right to use experimental drugs is Martin Delaney, a key player in the push to get the federal bureaucracy to provide that right.

Delaney is a man with an eclectic past. The son of a Chicago machinist, he entered a seminary and was close to being ordained a Jesuit priest before powerful doubts pulled him off that course. Later he became a successful businessman with a stable of corporate clients. His deft use of the media, a knack for negotiation, and the ability to inspire and train employees in the art of salesmanship were skills that served him well when he leaped into the AIDS drug fray.

Years earlier, Delaney had his own skirmish with the medical establishment. He had been diagnosed with chronic hepatitis and entered an experimental trial of two new drugs at Stanford University that hastened his recovery. That trial left him with permanent nerve damage to his feet—a common side effect of the drugs, which were soon abandoned as too toxic.

Not long after the therapies were pulled from further testing, Martin Delaney stood helplessly by as, one by one, five friends died from chronic hepatitis. Each suffered an untimely and painful death because no treatment was available. Delaney believes the choice to suffer nerve damage—and perhaps to live—should have been theirs to make.

In 1985, soon after his lover learned he was infected with the AIDS virus, Delaney helped found Project Inform, which is headquartered in San Francisco's Mission District. The organization was originally established to conduct community research and to monitor the progress of patients using unapproved medications. But that mission proved to be ahead of its time; no one was willing to fund it. Instead, Project Inform was restructured to help patients manage their own medical treatment. The organization began developing educational material about promising therapies, using strict medical criteria to select from among dozens of products pitched to AIDS patients.

Delaney fought publicly to peel away the FDA's many layers of consumer protection. "In the absence of approved options, whose interest is served by blocking access to partially proved remedies?" he asked. In the gray area between the preliminary promise of a drug and the moment it is ready to be approved, Delaney argued that "life-threatened patients and their physicians must have their hand-cuffs removed."

Activists like Delaney made a point of reminding the public that not all approved pharmaceutical products have turned out to be safe. DES (diethylstilbestrol), for example, was widely prescribed in the 1950s and 1960s to prevent miscarriages. More than fifteen years later, vaginal tumors linked to the drug were seen in the daughters of DES users.

More recently, a damning report issued by the General Accounting Office said that nearly half the new drugs approved for marketing in this country had severe or even fatal side effects that had not been identified during testing. Of 209 drugs approved for marketing be-tween 1976 and 1985, GAO investigators said 102 caused "serious" side effects. The FDA was furious with the report—Bob Temple, a top official in the agency's drug evaluation office, called it "garbage in, garbage out." Still, it helped expose the widely held myth that FDA approval automatically guaranteed the public's safety from dangerous drugs.

Many of the arguments advanced by patient advocates—that government officials should act faster, run fewer animal tests, be less concerned about drug side effects, and allow consumers and their physicians to decide what risks they want to take—paralleled those of ideological opponents to the whole drug regulatory process, the conservatives like Sam Kazman who believed the government should not poke its nose into the lives of its citizens at all.

"There is, to be sure, an incredible irony in all this," wrote Harold Edgar and David Rothman, two researchers at Columbia University. "Sick gay men, abandoned by a President who refused publicly to acknowledge their disease on all but one occasion, provided the shock troops to move forward his administration's deregulatory drug control program."

There was also a curious overlapping of interests with the pharmaceutical industry, which had long complained about the FDA's proclivity for caution at the expense of swift approval. Industry's motive was profit; the patient's motive was desperation. But the bottom line became the same—quicker access to new drugs. "Industry has always wanted to change the rules of the FDA," said Mathilde Krim, a scientist who led the charge to alter drug development norms. "The

activists provided industry a 'voice of the people.' They used each
other."

Politics does indeed make strange bedfellows.

Not everyone seconded the push to speed the availability of experimental products. In the absence of a cure for AIDS and in the face of
patient desperation, there were many vocal defenders of the FDA's
historic mission to keep dangerous or worthless agents off the shelves.

The search for effective AIDS treatments was characterized by
frequent fads and false hopes as the door opened wide to hucksters,
miracle makers, and quacks. Thousands of people with AIDS turned
themselves into human guinea pigs, theorizing they had little left to
lose. Word of promising therapies and magic potions spread like
wildfire, creating what was sometimes called the "drug-of-the-month
club." The rumor mill became a substitute for the prescription pad,
with a resultant free-for-all that advanced neither the cause of science nor patient health.

The FDA kept track of some of the quack scams. Not all of them
involved pharmaceutical products, but in every case outrageous medical claims were made. A mail-order operation did a thriving business
peddling bottles of processed T cells. A physician in the Caribbean
injected patients with cells extracted from the fetal tissue of pregnant
cows while another follower of the Hippocratic oath gave patients a
shot of their own urine. Other dubious remedies recorded by the FDA
include thumping on the thymus gland to stimulate the production of
white blood cells; bathing the body in chlorine bleach solution; and
exposing the genitals and rectum to the sun's rays at four o'clock
every afternoon.

It was hard to argue that the FDA should permit these and other
sham therapies to be marketed. Most agreed there had to be some
brakes on promoting and distributing unapproved therapies. Although the pendulum has swung closer to patient autonomy in recent
years, the focus of debate remains how best to apply those brakes.

Under a policy known as "compassionate use," the FDA had for
many years allowed desperate patients to use unapproved therapies
under certain circumstances, so long as they were not blatantly fraudulent. There were a number of ways unapproved drugs could be

secured. Often a doctor went directly to the drug company to plead for a supply of a promising new drug. Sometimes a patient's congressional representative would demand it. Whatever channels they used, seriously ill—but well-connected—individuals with access to good health care often had ways of getting drugs outside clinical trials.

Many thought the informal compassionate-use approach wasn't good enough. An enormous amount of paperwork was involved, long delays sometimes forced doctors to supply any drug they could get, rather than the one they actually wanted, and data was almost never collected on drugs distributed outside official studies. There were no well thought out, written procedures; the process had just evolved over time. "There were no meetings at FDA, no memoranda of meetings," said Peter Barton Hutt. "No one can recall a single group getting together at the FDA in the 1960s to talk about this. It was done primarily for humanitarian reasons. The doctors did this because it was good medicine."

Insiders at the FDA wanted to see the process formalized, and in the early 1970s there was a lot of talk about a system to make drugs that were being researched but had yet to be approved more widely available. Proposals were floated to link the final approval of a drug to the company's willingness to provide it for free first. Hutt hired a lawyer to write new regulations.

Then, in August 1974, scandal broke at the FDA. At hearings held by Senator Edward Kennedy, thirteen disgruntled employees charged that the FDA was so dominated by the pharmaceutical industry as to be ineffective. More investigations followed. For the next three years the FDA was consumed by its own internal probes and the need to open up shop to outside investigators, leaving little time for much else. Although the charges against the FDA were never substantiated, the resulting bottlenecks impeded innovation. As a result, all that really happened in the 1970s was the continuation of compassionate-use practices.

The issue refused to die. In the 1980s, scores of committees were formed—within the FDA, by congressional fiat, and under the auspices of the Pharmaceutical Manufacturers Association, the mouthpiece for the drug companies—to figure out better ways to make unapproved drugs available for therapeutic use. In 1983 the FDA proposed a set of broad regulations that would have made just about any investigational drug available to patients with serious illnesses.

It took four years to get a modified version of those regulations approved.

Meanwhile, the debate over expanded access to unapproved drugs was heating up. The conventional wisdom of scientists and regulators was being steered straight into a head-on collision with patients fighting for the right to make their own choices. It was the AIDS underground that first began to tip the scales of decision-making authority toward the gamblers. If the medical establishment was unable or unwilling to put drugs into their hands, smugglers and bootleggers, kitchen chemists, and bathtub *braumeisters* were going to do it instead.

4

THE AZT
BREAKTHROUGH

We have first raised a dust and then complain we
cannot see.

—BISHOP BERKELY,
*Principles of Human
Knowledge*

IN THE BRIEF HISTORY of AIDS drug development, the early 1980s
were bleak times. Three years after AIDS had been officially designated an epidemic by the federal Centers for Disease Control, 3,000
people had been diagnosed with the disease. And the death toll was
mounting.

The discovery of HIV had been cold comfort. Most scientists still
believed that retroviruses were inherently untreatable. The pharmaceutical industry was generally uninterested in AIDS because no one
thought the huge investment necessary to bring an effective drug to
market would pay off. Back then, corporate analysts were still dis-
missing the disease because it affected only a few thousand people.

Sam Broder thought differently. Broder was the son of working-
class parents, Jewish refugees who had fled war-ravaged Europe after
a long stay in a displaced person's camp. They had then run a diner
in Detroit, and had pushed their son hard to achieve something

better. Broder attended the University of Michigan as a scholarship student, developing the passion for science that helped launch his meteoric career. After completing his medical internship and residency at Stanford, he signed on with the National Cancer Institute, rising through the ranks as cancer ward physician, laboratory researcher, and eventually director.

Sam Broder has been one of the central figures in the struggle to find effective treatments against AIDS. Driven by compassion, foresight, and ambition, he became a cheerleader, aggressive and enthusiastic in his efforts to lead the government's response and to boost private sector involvement in research.

A Special Task Force on AIDS was established at the National Cancer Institute in 1984. Bob Gallo was scientific director, Sam Broder the task force's clinical director. Broder needed help. He was going to need more than his small staff and an 800-square-foot laboratory to develop a treatment for AIDS. The pharmaceutical industry had to get involved.

Hat in hand, Broder began knocking on doors across the country, making a plea to drug company officials. Broder was flying solo in those days. There had not been much interest from the upper echelons of the federal government's public health bureaucracy. No one else bothered trying to jawbone the drug companies into pursuing AIDS research. On his sojourns into the pharmaceutical hinterlands, Broder pledged to test promising compounds in NCI laboratories to see if they were effective against HIV. But he wanted something in exchange—a firm commitment to develop and market drugs that showed potential.

One of the companies Broder approached was Burroughs Wellcome, the American subsidiary of Wellcome PLC, a British-based conglomerate. Broder knew BW had worked with nucleoside analogues, the broad category of antiviral therapies that his honed scientific instinct told him might combat HIV, and had a record of accomplishment in viral research. Its success in bringing acyclovir—the first drug to prove effective against the herpes virus—to market convinced Broder that Burroughs Wellcome was well positioned to get involved in AIDS research.

At the time he was excited about initiating a dialogue with BW and hopeful that its corporate largesse and technical know-how could be used to advantage. Broder didn't have any personal connections at Burroughs Wellcome, but his colleague Dani Bolognesi, who was equally committed to AIDS, did know a few people. Bolognesi was working at Duke University Medical Center. Bolognesi made a few telephone calls and the stage was set for Broder to meet with some of Burroughs Wellcome's top scientists.

The first meeting took place on October 5, 1984, at company headquarters in the Research Triangle of North Carolina, a booming tricity area defined by the boundaries of Raleigh, Durham, and Chapel Hill, and anchored by computer firms and well-established universities. But if the region's economic prospects were good, early signals from Broder's autumn meeting with Burroughs Wellcome were not. At first the company turned its back on AIDS research.

One reason for this reluctance was the fear of working with live— and potentially fatal—AIDS viruses. Images of a haywire virus cutting a swath of death across the North Carolina laboratories haunted the dreams of BW scientists. One senior-ranking employee, in particular, knew from experience that such a vision was not confined to the pages of a science fiction thriller; he had watched helplessly as one of his colleagues died after being infected in the laboratory by a virulent virus he was studying. To be fully secure, HIV research had to take place in a highly controlled setting, termed a P-3 level of biosafety. Few labs in the research community were that safe, and the cost of readying one for HIV-related work was close to a quarter of a million dollars. Even for a company as large as Burroughs Wellcome, whose worldwide annual sales already exceeded a billion dollars, it was a sizable undertaking.

Such a commitment was especially formidable given the company's doubts that AIDS research could ever turn a profit. In one of the many ironies of the epidemic, Broder spent a lot of time that day convincing Burroughs Wellcome that an effective drug had commercial potential, that a reasonable return on investment could be secured. At first, corporate officials refused to budge. Broder finally flew off the handle at their indifference, insisting that AIDS was going to spread far beyond the 3,000 people who had already been diagnosed.

There is money to be made in AIDS, Broder said to Burroughs Wellcome. Perhaps big money.

Fear of working with the live AIDS virus was not restricted to drug companies. The NCI lab did not meet P-3 safety conditions either, but Broder felt he could not afford to wait until it was properly outfitted. Instead, he told his staff they were free to ask for a transfer. Many opted out. Hiroaki Mitsuya chose to stay.

Mitsuya, recruited by Broder from Japan because of his work on retroviruses, was a rising star who had already earned a medical degree and a doctorate in medical science from Kumamoto University. When Sam Broder first committed the National Cancer Institute to AIDS research, Mitsuya was earning less than $18,000 a year as a postdoctoral research fellow. Mitsuya turned his academic expertise on immune-system deficiencies to good use. He was the man who figured out an efficient, accurate, and safe way to screen compounds for their value against HIV. Mitsuya became, in Broder's words, "the best viral pharmacologist in the world, a one-person national resource."

Broder's persuasiveness, coupled with some coaxing from Bolognesi, eventually got Burroughs Wellcome to rethink its position on AIDS research. Along with fifty other drug companies, BW finally began shipping chemical compounds to NCI's lab to be tested for their effectiveness against HIV. Each sample was coded by letter to protect its identity—as well as the company's proprietary rights.

In February 1985, government researchers struck pay dirt. A drug shipped in by Burroughs Wellcome, and code-named Compound S, showed activity against HIV in the test tube. Apparently hoping to speed ultimate approval, Burroughs Wellcome also sent the compound to FDA laboratories for testing, but scientists there did not detect the same activity. Bolognesi and his colleagues at Duke University, however, did confirm the NCI finding.

Compound S was azidothymidine, also known as zidovudine, and soon to become known as AZT.

Broder had been on target with his hunch about nucleoside analogues, the class of drugs to which AZT belongs. The compound was not new. It was originally synthesized in 1964 by Jerome Horwitz, a researcher with the Detroit Institute for Cancer Research, with funding from the National Cancer Institute.

Like other scientists, Horwitz had been screening existing drugs to see if they held any value as cancer therapies. He became dissatisfied with that approach and soon turned to a more intellectually rigorous one—designing a compound specifically built to stop malignant cells from going berserk. AZT was the result of Horwitz's laboratory efforts. Unfortunately, it didn't work—there was no appreciable anti-tumor activity. But he was intrigued by the properties of AZT, whose main ingredient is thymidine, derived from the DNA in salmon and herring sperm. Instinct told him he had created a drug that would have to await the right disease to prove its value. But Jerome Horwitz never filed for a patent.

As a result, AZT remained in the public domain gathering dust until the 1970s. During that decade, scientists from the Max Planck Institute in Germany and from other research centers throughout Europe discovered that AZT was active against retroviruses in mice. By the early 1980s more studies had been published documenting the antiretroviral properties of AZT and related drugs in animals. Burroughs Wellcome tested AZT for veterinary applications, but chose not to develop it. No other commercial application was found. As far as scientists knew, retroviruses rarely caused disease in people, so the drug didn't seem worthy of further pursuit.

When the announcement came about AZT's effectiveness against HIV, scientists were cautiously optimistic. The drug appeared able to block the pathological changes that take place in infected helper-T cells and eventually destroys them, thereby exposing patients to life-threatening diseases. The hope was that by preventing viral replication, further damage to the immune system could be prevented, and ways might be found to restore the immune system to health. Especially good news about AZT was that it did not appear to affect DNA polymerase, an enzyme that catalyzes the making of normal DNA and also has a role in repairing damaged DNA. But scientists still adopted a wait-and-see attitude, knowing from long experience that the vast majority of drugs that produce good laboratory results prove ineffective, dangerously toxic, or both when administered to humans.

In June 1985, Burroughs Wellcome took the first formal step toward obtaining marketing approval for AZT when it submitted an application to the FDA for an Investigational New Drug (IND), which provides the protocol, or study design, to be used to learn about a drug's therapeutic value. Once the FDA approves an IND, the first phase of human testing can begin. During Phase I trials, a drug is tested on just a few people to ascertain its safety and to determine an appropriate dosage level; at this stage, the drug's effectiveness in treatment is secondary. Phase I studies scrutinize the drug's activity in the blood and spinal fluids.

If Phase I results look promising, researchers move on to Phase II to hone the proper dosage and find out how well a drug works, while continuing to monitor its safety. Phase III tests a drug for safety and effectiveness on a much larger body of patients. Traditionally, all three phases must be completed before a company can file a New Drug Application (NDA), the massive document the FDA requires to decide whether to approve a drug. (See Appendix B for a more detailed outline of the drug testing and approval process.)

The early reports about AZT were so enthusiastic—and the desperation to find an AIDS drug so intense—that an FDA committee gave the IND its blessing within the week. Thus officially sanctioned, Burroughs Wellcome, NCI, and Duke researchers were ready to proceed with their first Phase I study.

Eleven AIDS patients were recruited for the first phase of the historic AZT trial at NCI's own clinic facilities in Bethesda, Maryland. Eight more patients were enrolled at Duke University.

Typically, the corporate partner in a government/business collaboration does some of the analysis for Phase I studies. Broder had planned to send blood samples drawn from patients getting AZT down to North Carolina so that Burroughs Wellcome could test them. Days before the trial was scheduled to start, BW threw a wrench into the whole works when its officials announced they were backing out of that assignment. Once again, the nightmarish vision of a virus run amok had surfaced. Any sense of obligation to protect the health and safety of the American public had been overshadowed by fear at Burroughs Wellcome.

Broder remembered clearly the havoc caused by BW's eleventh-hour withdrawal. "We had a certain timetable, and speed was absolutely essential. Losing a couple of days was critical because a lot was riding on this," he commented. To keep the trial on track, Broder had to yank some people in his already strapped lab off another project.

On July 3, 1985, a furniture salesman from Boston became the first person ever to take AZT.

Within a few weeks, preliminary results from the Phase I trial were available—and they looked promising. Patients were able to absorb AZT, side effects were tolerable, and some clinical and immunological improvements were evident. But the trial still had months to run before researchers felt confident about the drug's safety.

Next came Phase II studies. Between February and June 1986, 282 people with AIDS or advanced symptoms of HIV infection were enrolled at twelve medical centers around the country. All but 13 were men. People with AIDS were required to have had a first episode of PCP (*Pneumocystis carinii* pneumonia) within the preceding four months, but to have had no other opportunistic infections. Those who had not been officially diagnosed with AIDS had to have unexplained weight losses, fungal infections, and at least one of a long list of other infections associated with the virus. Trial candidates were disqualified if they had recently used just about any other drug except aspirin, and even that required a researcher's permission.

Just six months into the trial, members of an independent monitoring board, who were privy to the data collected on all participants, were certain that patients on AZT were faring dramatically better than those on placebo—19 of the 137 patients on placebo had died, compared with just 1 of the 145 patients taking AZT.

On September 19, 1986, the blindfold was stripped from the trial, and all patients on placebo were offered the active drug.

Within a month, AZT was made available to some AIDS patients outside the trial on a compassionate-use basis while further testing continued. Between September 1986 and March 1987, BW gave away free AZT to some 4,500 people, or one-third of all those living with AIDS at the time. According to the company, the handouts cost $10 million.

The requirement for phase III studies was waived for AZT, a practice that is not uncommon when a life-threatening disease is involved. Instead of completing the last phase of the trials, BW buckled down to prepare its New Drug Application. Given the urgency of the need and the promise of the drug, the AZT application was submitted to the FDA in stages, beginning in October and ending on December 2, 1986.

Consistent with the rapid pace with which AZT had already rolled through the testing pipeline, FDA officials moved quickly to review the mountains of data in Burroughs Wellcome's application. There were grim reasons for the haste. As 1986 drew to a close, AIDS had claimed the lives of at least 23,000 Americans. Not one treatment had been approved. The FDA was under intense pressure to get a drug out.

Ellen Cooper was busy during that Christmas season. She had joined the FDA on a research fellowship in 1982. Her academic and medical credentials were impeccable—undergraduate work at Swarthmore, medical education at Yale and Case Western Reserve, a master's degree in public health from Johns Hopkins, and specialized training in pediatrics and infectious diseases. Everyone agreed that Cooper was a dedicated professional, a knowledgeable scientist, a top-flight researcher.

She also juggled more than an average share of family responsibilities, with four children—triplets and a youngster with Down's syndrome—to raise. Cooper's rise through the ranks of the FDA came swiftly. She was one of the first officials at the agency to become involved with AIDS drugs. When the FDA created the Division of Anti-Viral Drug Products to expedite its review of AIDS drugs, Cooper was chosen to head it. That position did not seem likely to place her solidly in the public eye. Ellen Cooper, after all, was a scientist, not a politician.

Circumstances, however, made her the point person for most of the FDA's early decisions about AIDS drugs. As a result, she found her judgments evaluated in a highly charged environment, and her reviews from FDA watchers were decidedly mixed. At times she became the target of rage and name-calling, bearing the brunt of some of the sharpest criticism levied against the FDA. But Cooper got high marks on AZT.

As others were drinking eggnog and making the rounds of tree-trimming parties, Cooper was performing yeoman's service. Day after day, night after night, she pored through Burroughs Wellcome's voluminous application. Her goal was to move AZT through the approval process as quickly as possible.

When Cooper had finished studying the AZT data, an FDA advisory committee was summoned to meet. The committee's job was to recommend to the FDA whether or not AZT should be approved. Usually, although not always, an advisory committee's recommendation on drug approval is followed to the letter.

The committee met just six weeks after Burroughs Wellcome had completed its application. The setting was the Parklawn Building in Rockville, Maryland, a bland glass box of a federal office building that is FDA headquarters. It is badly in need of a coat of paint and renovated elevators, and space is so cramped that the lounge in at least one women's rest room has been converted to an office. The building is an unmistakable symbol of the resource shortfalls that have long impeded the FDA's work.

One key question was on the table: Was AZT safe and effective enough to warrant the drug's approval? The answer would have far-reaching consequences.

Initially the debate suggested that data collected on the drug was insufficient. Over and over, committee members expressed grave concerns about the limitations of scientific knowledge about AZT and the fact that it had been tested during just one major trial lasting only six months. No one could say with certainty just who would benefit from AZT, or at what dose it should be administered. No one had determined whether the drug would remain effective over the long haul, or how toxic its side effects would prove to be.

Other doubts surfaced through the day. Committee members knew that even if the FDA approved the drug only for use by the narrow population in which it had been tested, physicians would make it much more widely available. Despite an absence of good data, Calvin Kunin, a committee member, observed that "once a drug is licensed, physicians do whatever they want to."

Ellen Cooper also expressed some reservations, warning, "Although we are all aware of the need for rapid clinical development of drugs to treat AIDS, the approval of a potentially toxic drug for marketing, particularly when it is anticipated that many less ill individuals will take it on a chronic basis, would represent a significant and potentially dangerous departure from our usual toxicology requirements."

There was talk about provisionally approving AZT and mandating further studies, but committee members agreed that it was hard to revoke a drug's license. "It is a fact of life that, once a drug is approved, it is almost impossible, as a practical matter, to withdraw that approval, unless there is a very serious safety consideration," said Edward Tabor, a high-level FDA manager.

At times the day-long meeting grew contentious, but in the end, the reservations that dominated the day's debate were set aside. By a ten-to-one vote, the committee gave thumbs-up to AZT.

Two months later, on March 19, 1987, the Food and Drug Administration accepted the committee's recommendation and approved the drug, clearing the way for any physician to write a prescription for its use by any patient. "For drug development," commented Sam Broder, "that is the speed of light."

SECOND THOUGHTS ABOUT AZT

Year after year, report after report, new drug after new drug, the AZT story has been touted as evidence that the testing and approval system can work. It was to be a model for the flood of therapeutic products expected to follow. And certainly there was much that was innovative about it.

Here was a public-private partnership in which the National Cancer Institute and a drug manufacturer worked in apparent harmony to test a promising compound quickly. Instead of passively awaiting Burroughs Wellcome's final application, the FDA followed the progress of the trials and reviewed available data at every step. The high-gear response to the drug allowed it to move from the IND stage to full marketing approval in less than two years, rather than the more typical eight years.

Anticipating approval, Burroughs Wellcome had disrupted production plans at several chemical plants and invested in new technology so that it could manufacture AZT in the necessary quantities. Right after the FDA okay, there were still shortages of the drug, largely because thymidine was hard to find—salmon and herring sperm weren't typically found on the shelves of most laboratories. Worldwide consumption of thymidine had long been stable at about twenty-five pounds a year, and the entire supply had been exhausted soon after AZT testing had begun. Fortunately, Pfizer developed a synthetic alternative to natural thymidine and began supplying it to Burroughs Wellcome. As a result, by the end of 1987, the drug was available in quantities sufficient to satisfy the explosive patient demand.

Despite these successes, fallout from the whole process was intense. AZT raised troubling issues that continued to surface as other promising drugs appeared on the horizon. Critics complained about the way the trial was designed and the fact that, in line with traditional scientific practice, the AZT Phase II study was conducted on a fairly homogeneous patient population—in this case, on gay white men. The goal was to limit variables that might distort the data.

That sounded reasonable—unless you were a drug user or a child with AIDS. Both groups were specifically excluded from access to the only drug that seemed to slow HIV. If you were a woman, getting on the Phase II AZT trial was extremely difficult—a total of thirteen women, less than 5 percent of the total number of participants, were enrolled. The exclusion of infected minorities and women, which began with AZT, continued for many years of AIDS drug research. As the demographics of the AIDS epidemic changed, that seemed steadily more discriminatory, spawned passionate complaint and even raised questions about the scientific validity of certain trials.

"The concept that good research, pure research, is color-blind begs the issue," said Janet Mitchell, a member of the board of directors of the National Minority AIDS Council. According to Dr. Mitchell, any study that failed to enroll population groups at risk for AIDS has not performed its job of assembling comprehensive data about a drug's value. "People are not specially bred laboratory specimens. Environment and culture can alter outcomes. . . . Research done in select populations cannot and should not be expected to produce results applicable to the general population."

Bitter questions were also asked about the astronomical price of AZT and eventually, about Burroughs Wellcome's right to its patent and to exclusive marketing rights. Some even questioned whether AZT worked at all.

5

PLACEBOS AND PROFITEERING

I got rich by honest graft. . . . I seen my opportunities
and I took 'em.

—GEORGE WASHINGTON
PLUNKITT,
Tammany Hall ward boss

DESPITE THE DOUBTS that later surfaced, most patients were initially
frantic to have a crack at AZT. Fueled by anecdotes and rumor, the
drug had developed "the status of a Holy Grail in the AIDS underground," according to Paul Monette in *Borrowed Time*, his moving
memoir of his lover's death. Admission into the AZT Phase II trial
often reflected political clout more than medical necessity. A telephone call from the White House to the National Cancer Institute got
at least one well-connected patient admitted.

Burroughs Wellcome was afraid that desperate patients might go
to desperate lengths, falsifying their medical records to qualify for the
AZT trial. To safeguard against such fraud, the company kept some
of its eligibility criteria under wraps. But other sub-rosa techniques
were used instead. Some AIDS patients offered cash to buy their way
into the trial; others extended bribes to BW employees who could
supply the drug. At company headquarters in North Carolina, AZT

was stored under lock and key, the tight security generally accorded only to narcotics.

The urgency with which patients demanded to join the first major AZT study highlighted issues that would echo time and again during the next few years: How could drugs be tested swiftly, and how soon could they be gotten into the hands of desperately ill people?

Mathilde Krim was one of the first people to leap into the debate. Krim was born in Italy and raised mostly in Geneva, Switzerland, where she grew up speaking Italian, German, and French. She traced the roots of her lifelong rebelliousness to the days immediately following the end of World War II, when she was a student at the University of Geneva. It was there that she learned the depth of Hitler's atrocities and was shocked to discover the intense anti-Semitism that still lingered.

Krim became fascinated with Judaic culture during her student years. Soon she was recruited as a courier for Irgun, the militant anti-British movement that helped establish the state of Israel, and she began running messages and weapons across international borders. In the early 1950s, she married David Danon, who was part of a circle of Zionist activists.

In 1953, with a newly earned doctoral degree from the University of Geneva, she moved with her husband and small baby to Israel. Her research career was launched at the Weizmann Institute of Science in Rehovot, where she studied genetics and cancer-causing viruses. Five years later, after a series of personal upheavals had turned her life around, she settled in an East Side town house in New York with her new husband, Arthur Krim, an attorney who later became chairman of Orion Pictures. Her scientific work continued at Cornell University and then at Memorial Sloan-Kettering Cancer Research Institute, where she headed the interferon laboratory.

Krim was in her late fifties when AIDS came along. As a biologist, she recognized the worldwide implications of a spreading infectious disease. The epidemic also brought back vivid memories of anti-Semitism. In her mind, the public attitude toward the gay community directly paralleled the attitude many Europeans had taken toward the Jews. In each case, those who were victims of oppression had gotten more blame than help; each group was accused of creating its own holocaust. Krim knew the devastating consequences of misplaced hostility and believed fervently that history could not be allowed to repeat itself.

In 1983, Mathilde Krim founded the first nonprofit organization to foster and support AIDS research. Little government money was available at the time, a reflection of the Reagan Administration's enraging indifference to the whole epidemic.

Two years later, Krim's organization merged with a similar one in California, which had been established by Michael Gottlieb, the UCLA researcher who struggled to keep Rock Hudson alive. From that synthesis was born the American Foundation for AIDS Research (AmFAR), the foremost private sponsor of AIDS research in the United States.

Until the AIDS epidemic forced a confrontation with the American biomedical establishment, placebo-controlled, double-blind trials were the gold standard of clinical research. In a placebo-controlled trial, half the patients received a medically useless "dummy" pill while the other half received an active drug. In a double-blind trial, neither the patients nor the investigators actually knew who was getting the active drug.

If no remedy, even an imperfect one, existed for a medical condition and there was no assurance that a new drug was safe and effective, placebos were an efficient research tool. But in a life-threatening situation they seemed terribly unfair, despite their time-honored value, because some sick and dying patients were forced to get a worthless drug.

Few people with AIDS fought to get on the AZT trial simply to further research. At a time when a climate of terror mingled with desperate hope in the patient community, the reason was understandably far less altruistic: they wanted a drug that might save their lives.

Mathilde Krim called placebos "morally unacceptable" in a life-threatening disease, and that was a common sentiment. Participation in the AZT study was time-consuming and risky. All patients had to be monitored regularly, journeying to trial sites to be poked and prodded and subjected to frequent blood tests and physical exams. They also had to swallow pills every four hours around the clock. And they were barred from taking additional medications without the approval of trial investigators. With a death sentence hanging over them, all those sacrifices seemed unfair just to get a chemically worthless pill.

"What is efficient for researchers can be deadly to study participants," said Mark Harrington, a New Yorker who championed the concept of giving patients a voice in drug research. Eventually the same cast of activist characters who strong-armed, sweet-talked, and badgered the power structure to change its other research and drug approval norms also challenged the placebo standard. In AIDS, anyway, that traditional pillar began to crumble.

Krim argued—first about the AZT trial, later broadening her argument to other drugs—that people who did not have time to wait were entitled to the most promising therapies available at the moment, even if neither safety nor effectiveness had been established with any certainty. She also spoke eloquently about the "unique and particularly cruel kind of torture" to which doomed patients felt subjected when they heard that a certain experimental drug "looked good," yet had no way to get it. In building the case that more people should have gotten AZT, either within the official trial or outside of it, Krim was not alone. Indeed, the eagerness with which patients sought that experimental drug established a recurring pattern.

Throughout the course of the epidemic, faint whispers about a promising new compound have engendered hope that sometimes bordered on hysteria. In response, the most well-connected people with AIDS—mostly gay, middle-class, white men—pushed aggressively to be research subjects. They followed reports about auspicious agents in newspapers, in the medical literature, and in underground newsletters, and monitored new drug applications to find out what the FDA was considering for approval. When a drug looked promising, they pulled out all the stops to get it. One researcher was offered a million dollars by a man desperate to enroll in his clinical trial.

From the groundbreaking AZT study to the present, patients also lied and cheated to be declared eligible for clinical trials. Some of the AZT trials were particularly plagued both by patient fraud and scientific carelessness. Word got out that the capsules containing AZT tasted different from the placebo, and a number of patients found out what they were taking before the discrepancy was corrected.

Anyone who missed that chance soon found another way to learn whether they were ingesting an active drug; they sent it to a laboratory and had its contents analyzed. In a rare display of patient solidarity, the data on AZT was further jeopardized when patients played a mix-and-match game, exchanging pills with one another to increase the odds of receiving the active drug.

Clinical investigators also had an opportunity to distort trial results. By the second week of treatment, routine blood counts of patients getting AZT looked different enough from those on the placebo that a careful observer could guess who was on the active drug. That meant that one of the cornerstones of traditional research—total objectivity—could not be assured.

The impact of those irregularities on AZT test results can never be calculated. How many patients had their drugs analyzed and made independent medical decisions on the basis of the answers? How many investigators actually noticed the change in blood count values and took mental note of them? Precise figures will never be known. Perhaps they had no meaningful impact on the study.

Or perhaps the effectiveness of AZT was so certain that a few distortions in the research did not alter the significance of the findings substantially. Certainly, numerous studies—conducted around the world to refine proper dosage levels and to compare its effectiveness to other drugs—later corroborated the finding that AZT prolongs life. The *New England Journal of Medicine*, for one, published a study in May 1991 that analyzed survival trends among AIDS patients. Those who took AZT after it was approved in March 1987 lived an average of 770 days; those who never took the drug after it was on the market survived only 190 days. Although the researchers could not say with absolute assurance that AZT was the sole reason, they concluded that "our data suggest that zidovudine (and perhaps other aspects of care associated with zidovudine therapy) has made a sizable difference in survival for persons with AIDS. . . . The challenge now appears to be to increase the use of that therapy in all segments of the population infected with HIV."

But experience has also demonstrated the limitations of AZT. At best, patients live only a few extra years. The drug commonly suppresses bone marrow, which causes anemia severe enough to require regular blood transfusions and forces the patient to stop treatment. Some researchers have also suggested a relationship between certain cancers and chronic use of the drug, especially in patients with advanced disease. And, alarmingly, AZT-resistant strains of the AIDS virus have been found in patients who have never even taken the drug.

The side effects and other medical restrictions have effectively barred almost half of the AIDS patient population from taking AZT. Some others, who were medically suited to the drug, became AZT "refuseniks." This faction—a vocal minority—was concentrated mostly in New York. Michael Callen was one of the leading voices of resistance.

Callen's AIDS diagnosis in 1982 had been the central demarcation point in his life. Before that, he had lived the promiscuous life of a man at loose ends, by his own admission substituting sex and drugs for meaning and commitment and getting by with occasional gigs as a cabaret singer. But after learning his grim medical diagnosis, Callen became a fighter. His own struggle for life was intense, but Callen turned his full powers on the government that consistently failed to respond adequately to the AIDS crisis. From the early days of the epidemic, Callen became locked in combat with members of the medical community who believed that AIDS was invariably terminal and that AZT was the best hope for prolonging life by a few years.

"Surviving AIDS is hard enough without attempting, at the same time, to survive AZT toxicity," wrote Callen in *Surviving AIDS*, his profile of patients who lived for years beyond their AIDS diagnosis.

The *New York Native* agreed with Callen's assessment that the antiviral medication had been distributed with unjustified abandon. "AZT is not a cure for AIDS," wrote John Lauritsen in an article published shortly after the FDA licensed the drug. "AZT's alleged benefits are not backed up by hard data, and are not sufficient to compensate for the drug's known toxicities. Recovery from AIDS will come from strengthening the body, not poisoning it. *Do not take, prescribe, or recommend AZT.*"

The merits and drawbacks of AZT continue to be hotly debated to the present day. While no unanimous consensus has emerged, most physicians and patients have continued to use the drug because they believe it is the best option available to them. Unfortunately, that is not saying much. And it speaks poorly for the whole drug testing system that tens of thousands of patients and their physicians have so few options to consider as they make their life-and-death decisions.

AZT's critics, however, tend to forget that the drug was never intended as a magic bullet against AIDS. It was only a good start, a breakthrough as significant psychologically as it was scientifically because it shattered the myth that retroviruses could not be stopped. This historical context has too often been lost.

Sam Broder, the man some called "Mr. AZT," wanted more than anything else to prove wrong the assumption that retroviruses were untreatable, although he knew the drug was no miracle cure. Looking back to the landmark days when AZT stood at the brink of approval, Broder said, "There is nothing magical or anointed about AZT. The key issue in that era, really my obsession, was to find something practical that would be shown at a clinical level to work. I felt the fate of all future antiretroviral drug development programs would be linked to the success or failure of AZT. If AZT succeeded, then many other programs would be possible. If AZT failed, it would set the field back many years."

Mathilde Krim agreed, remembering how reports of AZT had stirred hope within the scientific community. It suddenly seemed that AIDS might be recast as a treatable disease, not an inevitably fatal one. "When AZT came around, it became believable that something could be done about the virus," said Krim.

Sam Broder and Mathilde Krim, like many pharmaceutical companies, laboratory researchers, and AIDS patients themselves, assumed that a long line of more effective drugs would follow on the heels of AZT. It has not happened. Until October 1991, AZT was the only FDA-approved drug targeted directly at the heart of the disease—the AIDS virus itself.

And its cost was stunningly high.

THE PRICING OUTRAGE

Shortly before the FDA announced the approval of AZT, Burroughs Wellcome dropped a bombshell: the drug would cost patients as much as $10,000 a year, making it one of the most expensive prescription drugs in the nation's history.

A few weeks later, California Congressman Henry Waxman, who chaired the Subcommittee on Health and the Environment, held hearings to scrutinize the cost and availability of AZT. Subcommittee members grilled T. E. Haigler, then president of BW, at length, trying to establish his justification for the $10,000 price tag.

Haigler refused to be pinned down about actual research and development costs, instead speaking vaguely about the factors that went into the pricing equation. He said relevant considerations included "the costs of developing, producing, and marketing the drug, the high costs of research, and the need to generate revenues to cover these continuing costs." Also, according to Haigler, the company had factored in the uncertain market for AZT, the expected introduction of better therapies, and a margin for profit—just how wide a margin was anyone's guess. Finally, on the defensive, Haigler declared that sound business principles had been used to price AZT, concluding, "We didn't pick a number out of the air."

Still, Haigler's imprecise statements exasperated Ron Wyden, a Democratic congressman from Oregon. When he could restrain himself no longer, Wyden exploded. "Why didn't you set the price at $100,000 per patient?" he asked.

Haigler was startled by Wyden's outburst, but he recovered quickly and shot back, "I think that would have been completely out of the realm of anything reasonable at all. We had to set the price at a reasonable level."

Wyden continued to press Haigler. "I'm still unclear about how you arrived at $10,000 rather than $30,000 or $25,000. I appreciate your feeling that $100,000 is unfair. But I must tell you that I think the pricing system is close to a random system."

Burroughs Wellcome's strongest defense was its expectation that other antiviral medications would follow closely on the heels of AZT. Researchers and patients shared that sentiment, which meant the company had a year, two at the most, to recoup its research and development costs.

Haigler also claimed that AZT was costly to produce, noting that ten separate chemical reactions were required to create a synthetic

alternative to natural thymidine. An additional six steps converted
thymidine to AZT.

To meet the soaring demand for the drug, BW further alleged to
have poured $80 million into new technology and retooling so that it
could shift production plans at several chemical plants. In fact, that
$80-million figure was misleading, since a chunk of the money was
actually spent on the raw materials needed for future production,
rather than on the expenses of development. In any case, $80 million
is still less than the cost of developing the average drug, estimated at
between $90 and $231 million. Expenses were lower because drugs
typically take eight to ten years to get to market and require clinical
trials involving thousands of patients—but just two years had passed
from the time AZT was sent to Broder's lab until it was licensed by
the FDA. In the intervening time, only a few hundred patients were
enrolled in trials.

Perhaps the most galling aspect of the pricing issue was that AZT
was essentially a government drug. A reasonable principle of corporate investment is that the magnitude of profits should be related to
the extent of risk. Typically, a drug company is fully responsible for
the costs of preliminary research and drug development, with a lucrative payoff coming only if a compound is found to be safe and effective.

But AZT was financed very differently. In effect, the American
taxpayer footed the bill for the development and use of the drug at
least five times over. The first taxpayer dollars were funneled to
Jerome Horwitz, who originally synthesized the drug, through a grant
from the National Cancer Institute. Then more money came out of
public coffers when the drug was tested at NCI labs in the mid-1980s.
Next came government funding for Phase I clinical trials. The fourth
public subsidy was the liberal tax credits and exclusive marketing
rights given to BW for AZT under the terms of the Orphan Drug Act,
federal legislation passed in 1983 to encourage drug development for
rare diseases. Taken together, these breaks allowed the company to
write off as much as 70 percent of its clinical trial costs. And finally—
in the fifth use of government funds—Uncle Sam subsidized AZT for
patients who could not otherwise afford the drug. That meant that,
one way or another, Burroughs Wellcome could get its price and line
its pockets with the proceeds.

Whatever the blend of justification and profiteering behind the price of AZT, it brought BW a firestorm of criticism. Although the company announced a 20 percent price cut by the end of 1987, citing a drop in production costs, the $8,000-a-year price tag remained a thorn in the side of both the patient community and the public health establishment. A later price cut, again in response to public outrage, brought it down further, to $6,500, and reductions in the recommended dosage also made the drug more affordable. But none of that let Burroughs Wellcome off the hook.

In part because the government's role in the drug's development was so crucial, and partly because it was so expensive, Burroughs Wellcome and the National Cancer Institute bickered over who deserved credit for AZT.

AZT might never have been available had Sam Broder not prodded BW and encouraged collaborative efforts among investigators at the National Cancer Institute and Duke University. BW's contribution to early research was actually rather limited. Yet in its telling of the AZT story—in newspaper interviews, while under scrutiny at congressional hearings, in its annual report, and anywhere else it could get a forum—BW consistently airbrushed the government and academic scientists out of the picture. The reason was clear—base commercial interests. If BW amassed all the credit for inventing AZT, it could maintain the sole claim on the patent, and thus appropriate all the profits.

During Waxman's 1987 hearings, Haigler called the company's research into AIDS a "natural extension" of its antiviral program, which had gotten acyclovir to market. "This research began at a time when AIDS was not considered a significant public health problem by the general public, and pharmaceutical manufacturers generally did not consider the illness to be one involving significant financial rewards," said Haigler.

He then traced the company's AIDS research efforts back three years. But his account on Capitol Hill that day was rife with omissions. Haigler said, "In November 1984, we identified a compound, AZT, also known as azidothymidine or zidovudine, and which we now call Retrovir, which inhibited the replication of certain animal viruses in the laboratory."

He did not, however, admit that earlier researchers had paved the way. Not a word was spoken about the German researcher Wolfram Ostergag, who had published that same finding a decade earlier.

Furthermore, according to the company president, "independent laboratory testing in late 1984 and 1985 confirmed that zidovudine was effective in inhibiting multiplication of the human AIDS virus in the test tube." Actually, the independent laboratory testing—conducted at NCI—did not *confirm* the effectiveness of AZT against the AIDS virus, but identified it for the first time. Hiroaki Mitsuya rightfully deserved most of the credit for those early lab experiments—and it was his name that appeared as first author when the findings were published in the October 1985 *Proceedings of the National Academy of Science*. BW did not even corroborate NCI's findings because it had neither the facilities nor the courage to work with live AIDS virus.

Sam Broder was incensed by Haigler's testimony before the Waxman committee. In a private letter dated March 19, 1987, to David Barry, BW's vice-president of research, Broder clarified NCI's contribution to the development of AZT and blasted the company for its public posturing.

"From your recent testimony before the Waxman committee, the position of the Burroughs Welcome Company would appear to be that AZT was developed within the company with little substantive contribution by others," wrote Broder. "Your position saddens me and my colleagues at the National Cancer Institute, and strikes at the very heart of my ability to collaborate with you. . . . We need reciprocity here."

Broder also issued a stern warning to Burroughs Wellcome, writing that future projects with the federal government would be jeopardized if the company continued to claim the lion's share of the glory.

Broder's quiet diplomacy failed to silence the company. Over the next two years, in public forums and corporate publications, BW continued to boast of its solo role in the discovery of AZT. The company's exclusive hold on AZT also allowed it to manipulate AIDS research. If Burroughs Wellcome officials "didn't want the drug tested in a particular clinical trial," admitted one high-ranking government official at the time, "that clinical trial would not take place."

No one could have guessed how long BW's greedy grip on AZT

would last. Rival drugs never arrived to cut sharply into sales. In 1989, $225 million worth of AZT was sold, more than 40 percent above the previous year. By the end of 1991, cumulative sales of the drug exceeded $1 billion. Even with the approval of ddI in 1991—and the likelihood that ddC was not far behind—AZT has remained one of the prime weapons in the defense against AIDS.

6

THE RISE OF THE AIDS UNDERGROUND

❖

All together, we beat down the doors of the system and made it take our count. Some have sat in medical libraries wading through the arcana of immunology. Others pass back and forth over the border, bringing vanloads of drugs the law hasn't got around to yet. . . . If the government was going to act as if we didn't exist, if the medical establishment was prone to gridlock over funds, if the drug companies were waiting till the curve got high enough for profit, then we would find our own way. Whistling in the dark is whistling still.

—PAUL MONETTE,
*Borrowed Time: An AIDS
Memoir*

MARCH 1987 was a demarcation point in the history of AIDS drug development. Events within the world of AIDS were lively and sometimes bizarre. The approval of AZT seemed to unleash a potent force into the world. Patient empowerment—the refusal to be passive victims, the insistence on fighting the system that would pronounce their doom, the willingness to take matters in their own hands—became a reality. That influence shaped the policy response to AIDS and eventually inspired broader changes as advocates for people with Alzheimer's, breast cancer, schizophrenia, and other diseases began to approach their diseases with new militancy.

Within the few short weeks of March, a business partnership was formed that evolved into a "guerrilla" drugstore; the AIDS Coalition to Unleash Power (ACT UP), which would become an angry, loud, and highly effective political pressure group, held its first meeting; and the FDA stepped forward with a daring plan to get drugs into patients' hands before they had been approved. Over the next several years, each one of these milestones dramatically altered the course of the nation's response to the AIDS epidemic.

SMUGGLING RINGS

The man from San Francisco rang a friend in San Diego and asked, "Is it sunny in Tijuana?"

"No," came the response, "it's a cloudy day."

To an outsider, it would have sounded like a straightforward weather report. But the conversation had a broader significance—the callers were part of an elaborate smuggling network and they were communicating via a prearranged code. Their contraband—unapproved pharmaceuticals thought useful for treating AIDS. When the sun was shining, it meant drugs were plentiful and operators could bring sought-after medicines up from Mexico, beginning the process of putting them into the hands of thousands of patients. A cloudy prediction meant the mission would have to be postponed for the moment.

Drug trafficking began months before the first human trials on AZT, and continues to this day. The initial impetus for the elaborate bootleg operations were medical journal reports about the promise of ribavirin, a multipurpose antiviral medication that had been studied for twenty years before AIDS, and of isoprinosine, which was believed to bolster the immune system. In this country, neither product could be secured outside clinical trials, which inched along painstakingly and inconclusively.

In Mexico, though, ribavirin and isoprinosine were both sold over the counter—walk in with American dollars, a currency preferred to the sagging peso, walk out with drugs. No prescription was necessary. Word soon spread about willing suppliers in the border towns of Tijuana and Ciudad Juárez. Mexican pharmacies even advertised their drugs in gay publications in San Francisco and Los Angeles. Some included "clip-and-save" coupons offering special discounts.

Although no one tallied the numbers of people making the journey south of the California and Texas state lines, many Mexican drugstores were unable to keep either ribavirin or isoprinosine in stock for long. As demand soared and the Mexican economy floundered, some pharmacies tripled their prices for both drugs. Meanwhile, people with AIDS became increasingly systematic in their approach to securing them. Consumers organized to negotiate huge price breaks for quantity purchases. Some talked about setting up a large-scale distribution network on the California side of the Mexican border. One highly informed writer who called himself "Tooth Fairy"—and who years later was revealed to be Martin Delaney—began leaving advice about successful smuggling techniques under the pillows of San Francisco activists.

At about the same time, Delaney was launching Project Inform in San Francisco. One of its first official acts was to issue a detailed guide to running drugs up from Tijuana. With blow-by-blow precision, the document described the best routes to town and the *farmacias* most likely to carry ribavirin and isoprinosine. It even offered practical advice about how to dress, suggesting that fashions associated with the "gay look" be left in the closet. "Wear your least noticeable earrings, or none at all," advised the Project Inform document. "Leather gear can also be left at home or at least kept under your clothing."

Ways to avoid detection by U.S. Customs inspectors were also described in the Project Inform document. The most cautious approach was to bring back very small quantities of drugs, since the FDA unofficially allowed individuals to carry unapproved medicines for their own personal use. The drawback to caution was the need to shuttle frequently back and forth to Mexico.

The "smuggler samaritan" strategy was a popular alternative, adopted, according to Project Inform, by people who "choose to answer to a higher authority." Smuggler samaritans concealed large quantities of illegal drugs inside spare tires, wrapped them in clothing, stowed them under car floor mats, or squeezed them into ash-trays. To blend inconspicuously with the crowds of Americans who crossed the border to shop, buy cheap liquor, and get a taste of a foreign land, they typically dressed like tourists and "family men," often wearing polyester golf slacks or dangling cameras conspicuously. At least one man asked a pregnant woman to travel with him, hoping to ease the suspicion of border authorities.

For months, Customs and the FDA essentially ignored the drug traffic. But in May 1985 the bootlegging network generated a flurry of unwanted press attention, and Customs officials took action. While knowing the answer perfectly well, Customs made a show of asking the FDA whether ribavirin and isoprinosine were legal drugs. When the FDA said no, they began to confiscate them.

An outcry followed. By summer the policy had been reversed and the FDA agreed that people carrying small amounts of ribavirin or isoprinosine into the United States should be left alone. But the FDA was deliberately vague, and no one knew exactly how much of the drug would be allowed in. And it was another three years before the FDA would loosen up further and allow importation by mail.

Meanwhile, buyers' clubs appeared on the scene.

BUYERS' CLUBS AND AL-721

Buyers' clubs started trafficking in a food product known as AL-721, a butterlike concoction that derived its name from the ratio by which three active lipids extracted from egg yolks were blended together—seven parts to two parts to one part. Developed by cancer researchers at the Weizmann Institute of Science in Israel, AL-721 had already proved valuable in treating patients with age-associated memory loss and in easing the withdrawal symptoms that drug addicts and alcoholics experience during detoxification.

AL-721 took center stage in November 1985, when Robert Gallo and other researchers published a letter in the *New England Journal of Medicine* suggesting that AL-721 might inhibit the AIDS virus. The drug altered the structure of the T-cell membranes, so that when HIV zoomed in, it became destabilized and was unable to bind to the membrane. AL-721 had no apparent side effects and Gallo recommended further study of the drug. When his letter appeared, AZT was only a speck of hope on a distant horizon. Few other drugs even looked promising. Not surprisingly, AIDS patients and their advocates got excited.

The patent for AL-721 was held by Ethigen, a tiny company in Beverly Hills then called Praxis Pharmaceuticals. Because it was actually a food product, the manufacturer was legally permitted to sell it without restrictions, so long as no medical claims were made. Ethigen chose instead to pursue FDA approval for AL-721 as a prescription drug.

Bottom-line considerations were the obvious reason. The egg lipids were the only product for sale when the company went public. The opening price for stock shares was $1.25. Ten months later, when the Gallo letter appeared, the price more than tripled, to $4 a share. By pumping up investor excitement over the prospect of an upcoming AIDS drug, Ethigen was able to spur $3.7 million in stock sales, a sum it could never have attracted to market a nutritional supplement. The value of the strategy was confirmed after a tiny clinical trial showed promise; when the results became known, stock shares shot up to $11.

A few people traveled to Israel for AL-721 and wrote back glowing testimonials about its effectiveness. The patient community watched and waited for further studies. But researchers were otherwise engaged.

While the waiting continued, the first issue of *AIDS Treatment News* *(ATN)* was published by John James, a tall, gangly writer who remains a key player in the sophisticated network of AIDS drug information. James, who works from an overcrowded, paper-packed office in a nineteenth-century Victorian building in San Francisco, is self-taught; once a computer programmer, he had neither medical training nor a scientific background when he launched the newsletter. That didn't stop him from publishing a must-read monthly that patients often use to introduce new remedies to their own physicians. Along with patients, regular subscribers include government officials, drug companies, and members of the media. To this day, *ATN* investigates whispered rumors of new drugs, sheds light on alternative therapies, and lobbies for expanded access to experimental products.

In an early issue of his newsletter, James called AL-721 a promising treatment that had fallen "victim to a public policy nightmare of bureaucratic and commercial red tape." His interest in the drug helped convince others of its value, and soon recipes for AL-721 were being printed in gay publications across the nation. People began improvising bizarre concoctions brewed in their own kitchens, although no one knew whether simulated AL-721 was as good as the original product.

Worse, making home brews of the drug could be dangerous business. To extract the necessary ingredients, a solvent such as acetone was sometimes boiled with the egg yolk, and several people perished in flash fires when this mixture exploded. A random check of bootleg manufacturers also turned up widespread microbial contamination. Clearly, home kitchens couldn't replace the laboratory.

But many people remained enthusiastic about AL-721. In the pivotal month of March 1987, a group of New Yorkers with AIDS formed a business partnership with the aim of putting a more consistent AL-721 substitute into the hands of those who wanted it. To assure quality control, they even contracted with a laboratory to test each batch for bacterial contamination and to verify its chemical composition.

The decision to develop and distribute an AL-721 substitute opened the door to a possible suit from Ethigen on the grounds of patent infringement. But the company took no legal action. Ironically, the proliferation of copycat products instead prompted the company to market AL-721 as an over-the-counter nutritional supplement after all. Ethigen never did get any clinical trials off the ground, and eventually its interest in AL-721 waned. By then the scientific community had AZT, and financing for a fledgling company touting an egg derivative as a cure for AIDS was hard to nail down.

That did not deter the underground egg lipid business, however, which took off like a shot. A year after it was formed, the New York business partnership was generating $1 million in receipts.

It soon became apparent that egg lipids had little impact on the disease, and sales dwindled. But that early business partnership evolved into the People With AIDS Health Group, still based in New York City, which became the largest of dozens of guerrilla drugstores around the country.

Buyers' clubs operate in a shadowy twilight zone somewhere be-

tween a licensed drugstore and a pharmaceutical Casbah. Most sell
vitamins, minerals, and other over-the-counter products at bargain-
basement prices, but their principal business has been drugs that are
otherwise unavailable in this country. That is where buyers' clubs
move well into the gray zone that separates legal activities from
illegal ones.

The PWA Health Group is headquartered in New York's Chelsea
district, once a manufacturing center and more recently a hub of
publishing activity, cavernous dining spots, billiard parlors, and late-
night discotheques. In its cramped fourth-floor offices, a chalkboard
lists the prescription and over-the-counter drugs for sale. Many are
unavailable elsewhere. Orders are filled on the spot or shipped out by
mail. Payment options show just how sophisticated these underground pharmacies have become; American Express, MasterCard,
and VISA are all accepted. Although it has only a handful of employees and an annual budget of about $100,000, sales are far from
minuscule. In 1990, some $400,000 in goods were sold; in both of the
two years before that, when the club was trafficking in more expensive pharmaceuticals, receipts totaled $1 million.

In San Francisco, the Healing Alternatives Foundation has much
the same feel. HAF was born at the Metropolitan Community
Church in the Castro neighborhood, a progressive ecumenical institu-
tion with strong ties to the gay community. At church-basement
meetings, people came to share rumors and recipes for homemade
potions. John James was often there to offer his up-to-the-minute
insights about promising therapies. The excitement sometimes bordered on bedlam as speakers barraged the audience with information
and responded to the rapid-fire questions shot at them. The thrust of
the discussion was generally the same: How can we get our hands on
drugs rumored to be effective?

Soon the Healing Alternatives Foundation took organizational
shape to help people with AIDS do just that. It settled into the second
floor of a building on Market Street, the city's main thoroughfare, a
few doors down from a Libertarian bookstore. An acupuncture clinic
rents space in the same building.

Inside HAF offices, a staff member can often be found measuring
quantities of powder onto a scale. Another handles behind-the-
counter sales to buyers who come in clutching physicians' prescrip-

tions for unapproved medicines. Aloe vera juice, garlic capsules, and vitamins and minerals of all descriptions are also offered for sale. Along with its pharmaceutical cornucopia, the buyers' club serves as a clearinghouse for information about HIV and has a treatment library. A chilling reminder of the brutal realities of AIDS are index cards posted on a bulletin board—many announcing the sale of drugs collected from the medicine cabinets of people who have recently died.

At first glance, casual visitors cannot tell whether they have walked into an aboveboard pharmacy or an illicit drug den.

Buyers' clubs evolved partly to safeguard the health and pocketbook of a desperate community; most remain very selective in what they choose to sell. If a drug is likely to have serious side effects, most clubs won't handle it. They also stay away if a drug is unreasonably expensive, if there is reason to suspect fraud, or if the product seems likely to raise people's hopes pointlessly. Over the years, many drugs have been added to the underground medicine chest. But one of two key questions is always asked first, according to Derek Hodel, head of the PWA Health Group: Are the benefits so great that the toxicity is manageable? Or: Is the toxicity so negligible that even a theoretical benefit is worthwhile?

The clubs pride themselves on responding to demand rather than creating it. "The thrust of the buyers' clubs is empowerment," said Lewin Usilton, president of the board of the Healing Alternatives Foundation, whose long white hair and flower-patterned shirt suggest a kinship with Timothy Leary, a comparison he resists. "We're not here to push products, but there are a lot of people who are desperate."

At first, importing drugs was an administrative nightmare. Everything had to be learned by trial and error. "We hadn't any idea of what it meant to go through Customs," Hodel complained.

Today, importation has become almost routine. The way the PWA Health Group imports its drugs is fairly typical. Chemicals of hope are secured through scores of international connections. "The Health Group has spies all over the world. And we need more," proclaimed its newsletter in May 1990, calling for new volunteers in Europe, Israel, Australia, South Africa, Asia, and South America. "We need people on whom we can call at a moment's notice, who might be willing to run some errands," said the newsletter, deliberately vague about the precise nature of the volunteer mission.

In Dallas, one patient even maneuvered his way through the elaborate Mexican bureaucracy, making the necessary payoffs to public officials and ending up with a druggist's license that allows him to purchase compounds from wholesale distributors. "If you are well enough plugged in or smart enough or just ballsy enough, you can get anything you want," said Hodel.

Overseas orders are grouped together to get bulk prices and to save on shipping costs—once fifty or a hundred orders come in, buyers contact pharmacies in several countries to find out about current prices and to confirm a drug's availability. When necessary, a translator participates in a conference call to complete the negotiations. Private courier services are generally used to carry packages across international borders. The club handles all the customs documentation, pays the necessary tariffs, and has become expert in the arcane world of international currency fluctuations.

And yet Derek Hodel felt no sense of triumph as buyers' clubs became an effective, accessible source for drugs. Rather, he was disappointed by the failings of the medical establishment. "The underground has become mainstream and this is inexcusable," he said. "The majority of my clients and their physicians are not activists; they are simply desperate and have worked the system to the point of no return. They come, having already made the twentieth or thirtieth phone call trying to locate a trial for which they will qualify. No one approaches the underground as a first choice. They come because they have no other reasonable options."

THE FDA RESPONSE

At first the buyers' clubs and the smugglers seemed certain to test the limits of FDA tolerance. "We're treading on the edge of liability," admitted Lewin Usilton. But the regulatory agency was startlingly lax in its response. When they began distributing AL-721, for example, members of the PWA Health Group were prepared to be arrested. "We imagined the FDA would appear with guns drawn," said Derek

Hodel. But not much ever happened then—or later, when they turned their attention to fluconazole.

Fluconazole is used in the treatment of cryptococcal meningitis, an inflammation in the lining of the brain, caused by a yeastlike fungus usually found in bird excrement. The disease, which affects the central nervous system and is often fatal, is by far the most common fungal infection associated with AIDS. Fluconazole seemed a promising substitute for amphotericin-B, a drug with horrendous side effects, including flulike symptoms, vomiting, kidney toxicities, and anemia. The drug, known to patients as "amphi-terrible," is, not surprisingly, difficult to tolerate for long periods. Fluconazole represented the buyers' clubs' first foray into the murky waters of prescription drug importation. Until then they had handled only over-the-counter products. But in March 1989 the PWA Health Group decided to challenge FDA authority even more explicitly by setting up an overseas network of doctors and pharmacists to help fill American prescriptions for unapproved drugs. It was not a hidden venture; the buyers' club went public with its plan at a press conference called that month.

Soon physicians, including many who practiced only mainstream medicine, began knocking at the door of the PWA Health Group to request the drug for their patients. For almost a year, until fluconazole won FDA approval, the PWA Health Group was almost the only place outside clinical trials where the drug could be secured. Pfizer, the corporate sponsor, actually made the drug available to physicians on a compassionate-use basis but the program was mostly kept under wraps and few people knew of its existence.

The FDA was concerned enough about the challenge to its authority to request a meeting with the buyers' club's top brass—but it allowed imports of fluconazole to continue unhampered.

The Healing Alternatives Foundation had a similar experience with the FDA. Just once, an inspector poked around HAF offices for four days, snapping photographs of everything the club was selling. But after that spurt of activity, the inspector merely asked for a few labeling changes.

Why did the FDA keep such a low profile? In part, the decision not to crack down on activities of questionable legality reflected the agency's long-standing tradition of responding compassionately to the needs of desperate patients. Resource shortfalls also had an impact on the agency's ability to do its job. At the time, a third reason may have been the most decisive: with the shortage of approved products to treat AIDS, the FDA simply couldn't afford the political liability of clamping down. But there was no assurance that the FDA would stay forever at arm's length from the buyers' clubs. In the early 1990s, when a new commissioner came on board pledging stricter law enforcement, the clubs got nervous—although not nervous enough to stop doing what they had gone into business to do.

7

ACTIVISM, ACT UP, AND DEXTRAN SULFATE

And ill it therefore suits
The mood of one of my high temperature
To pause inactive while awaiting
Of desperate cure for those so desperate ill.

—THOMAS HARDY,
The Dynasts

JAMES CORTI'S KNACK for tracking down sought-after drugs made him something of a legend in underground circles. Corti, a registered nurse, bicycle racer, and painter from Los Angeles, was moved by personal tragedy to get involved. He began trafficking in underground drugs soon after his lover died from AIDS, cutting his teeth on the Mexico-to-United-States ribavirin caper.

In a business that had its share of unethical practitioners, Corti was an honest man. Typically, he would start an import network but turn it over to others to run. Then he watched with a hawk's eye to spot profiteers. From time to time he jumped back into the business to undercut a greedy salesman by peddling a drug at cost. "Jim Corti is the one who cuts the profit out of the AIDS underground," claimed Martin Delaney.

It was dextran sulfate that earned Corti much of his early notoriety—and the nickname "Dextran Man." Interest in dextran sulfate to treat AIDS dated back to the summer of 1986. Donald Abrams, a well-known AIDS researcher at San Francisco General Hospital, was contacted at the time by Ryuji Ueno, a Japanese scientist whose father owned Ueno Fine Chemicals Industry in Osaka.

Abrams, himself a gay man who later lost a lover to AIDS, had been a part of inner scientific circles since the epidemic's early days. Abrams was impressed by Ueno's laboratory data, which suggested dextran sulfate might work against HIV by inhibiting the binding of the virus to the surface of the T cell. Dextran sulfate also had a second mode of attack, apparently preventing the cell-to-cell attack in which infected T cells turn on healthy ones.

The researchers were especially interested in the possible benefits of using dextran sulfate in combination with AZT. Abrams agreed to run a Phase I trial. To attract patient enrollment, Ueno published a letter in *The Lancet*, the British medical journal, in which he hinted about dextran's promise. That letter set in motion a series of events that made the scientists sorry they had ever sought publicity.

The *Lancet* letter immediately attracted patients' attention. While Abrams was beginning his FDA-sanctioned trial, word spread through the patient communities across the United States that dextran sulfate was widely available over the counter in Japan. The product had been developed in the 1960s to treat arteriosclerosis and to lower cholesterol levels. In another form it was also used with blood transfusions to minimize clotting. Dextran sulfate was generally believed to be safe. It was also cheap; AZT cost some $800 a month when it was first approved, while the standard dosage of dextran ran about $1,000 a year.

Demand soared. A bootleg distribution system was put in place. James Corti was one of its masterminds. He dealt mostly in cash, walking into a Tokyo pharmacy with a brown paper bag filled with yen and walking out with tens of thousands of dollars' worth of the white dextran sulfate tablets. Then he'd ship out packages marked as Japanese dolls and tea sets in order to move them past the watchful eyes of Customs officials.

Many flight attendants and American expatriates living in Tokyo soon had second careers—as smugglers. With their help, Corti and others managed to bring some $2 million worth of the drug from

Japan into the United States. Most of it was funneled to eager AIDS patients through buyers' clubs around the country.

Not everyone was happy about the booming import business. For one thing, the availability of illicit dextran sulfate allowed trial participants to supplement their official dose with drugs obtained on the street. An anonymous letter sent to Abrams by a man who was not enrolled in the study, but was buying dextran sulfate from someone who was, alerted him to the irregularities that riddled his trial.

"I understand from my friend in your study that several participants are not taking the doses you think they are," claimed the man. "I am hoping your test results will in some way reflect this erroneous input. Would a lie detector test be helpful?"

Nor were the Japanese thrilled about the large-scale exportation of dextran sulfate. Ueno Fine Chemicals was disgruntled at the possibility of losing exclusive access to the lucrative market in the United States. The Japanese government was alarmed at the likely influx of HIV-infected Americans traipsing through their country in search of drugs. Without warning, they clamped down on the sales of dextran sulfate for export.

Although a chemically identical drug was manufactured by fourteen different Japanese pharmaceutical companies, Kowa Pharmaceutical's product had somehow become the brand of choice. The scuttlebutt was that either the Japanese or the American government had pressured Kowa to cut off the supply to retail distributors. The Japanese continued to have access to dextran sulfate, as before, but in the spring of 1988, Americans were shut out. For a brief time, opportunistic Japanese businessmen stepped in to fill the void, purchasing tablets in huge quantities and adding a markup on every pill they resold. For a few hours' work, these middlemen were pocketing up to $30,000 in profits.

People who had raced to Japan for dextran sulfate felt desperate. Something had to be done.

SILENCE EQUALS DEATH

ACT UP was born on March 10, 1987, in the basement of the Lesbian and Gay Community Services Center on 13th Street in Greenwich

Village. Nora Ephron was scheduled to talk, but canceled at the last
minute, and Larry Kramer was asked to step in.

In public, Kramer has a reputation as a bit of a loose cannon; some
of his outbursts are legendary. In one forum he called Tony Fauci,
director of the National Institute for Allergy and Infectious Diseases
and head of the government's principal AIDS research effort, a "monster." On another occasion he said, "Almost every person connected
with running the AIDS show everywhere is second-rate." Kramer has
also charged the federal government with genocide, and before the
Sixth International AIDS Conference in San Francisco, in 1990, he
had reached such a level of frustration that he called openly for
terrorism. Although he admitted later, in a private interview, that he
hadn't really expected activists to throw bombs or conduct sabotage,
he continued to believe it was the only way to bring the needed sense
of urgency to AIDS. "We're such good little boys," Kramer said.
Hearkening back to the underground movement that helped create
the State of Israel, he asked, "Where is our Irgun?"

His private persona is very different. In the relative seclusion of his
two-bedroom apartment overlooking Washington Square Park,
Kramer seems just as intense but a lot more introspective. From his
window, the Village explodes with its unique brand of *joie de vivre*.
On a typical spring day, the park is thick with jugglers, unicyclists,
singers, and wide-eyed college students mixing in apparent harmony
with soccer-playing Rastafarians, skateboard enthusiasts, residents
on jaunts with their pet boa constrictors, chess players, drug dealers,
and ordinary folks. But the deaths of literally hundreds of friends and
professional associates and his own HIV-positive status have not allowed Larry Kramer to view his backyard with much joy. In private,
it is easy to sense the suffering he has witnessed, the grief that
underlies his public rage.

One thing about both the public and the private Larry Kramer: he
is a man who seldom hesitates to speak his mind. Kramer accepted
the short-notice invitation to speak at the local community center that
wintry March night.

After looking over his audience of 250 people, he asked about
two-thirds of them to stand. When they had, he delivered this grim
prognosis: "At the rate we are going, you could be dead in less than
five years. If my speech tonight doesn't scare the shit out of you, we're

in real trouble. If what you're hearing doesn't rouse you to anger, fury, rage, and action, gay men will have no future here on earth. How long does it take before you get angry and fight back?"

Kramer went on to criticize Gay Men's Health Crisis for devoting insufficient energy to political lobbying and advocacy—the New York group was always more focused on patient services—and pleaded for stronger leadership:

> I want to talk to you about power. We are all in awe of power, of those who have it, and we always bemoan the fact that we don't have it. Power is little pieces of paper on the floor. No one picks them up. Ten people walk by and no one picks up the piece of paper on the floor. The eleventh person walks by and is tired of looking at it, and so he bends down and picks it up. The next day he does the same thing. And soon he's in charge of picking up the paper. And he's got a lot of pieces of paper that he's picked up. Now—think of those pieces of paper as standing for responsibility. This man or woman who is picking up the pieces of paper is, by being responsible, acquiring more and more power. He doesn't necessarily want it, but he's tired of seeing the floor littered. All power is the willingness to accept responsibility. But we live in a city and a country where no one is willing to pick up pieces of paper. Where no one wants any responsibility. . . .
>
> Well, until we all bend over and pick up all those little pieces of paper, I don't have to tell you what's going to happen.

Two days after Kramer's pleas, several hundred people met again and began to fight back in earnest. The new organization was christened ACT UP, and soon afterward a logo was adopted—the despised pink triangle worn by homosexuals in the concentration camps of Hitler's Germany. But this time the gay community declared its refusal to be victimized—the triangle points up and bears a grim motto: "Silence = Death."

ACT UP's ground rules require the organization to function without a board of directors, paid staff, or elected leader. Control of the floor is assigned to a "facilitator" who changes regularly. Anyone can vote after attending two sessions—but since no one takes attendance, it is impossible to know whether that restriction is respected.

On a typical Monday night, 400 ACT UP members will crowd into

Cooper Union's Great Hall on Astor Place, the dividing line between East Village and West Village. The weekly town meeting has been variously described as a bold experiment in participatory democracy and an exercise in creative chaos. The agenda is lengthy, with everyone in the audience allowed to comment on every issue. Meetings run upwards of five hours, and many dedicated members also attend one or more of the twenty-plus committee meetings that are held every week.

Over the years, ACT UP's name and tactics have been adopted by numerous groups around the country as well as in Europe, Australia, and Canada. Activists mastered the art of the sound bite, the thirty-second quotable tidbit so well loved by television news reporters. They also pioneered telephone and fax "zaps," in which the lines of target agencies are jammed with hundreds of simultaneous calls, and they have even received an award for street theater from New York City's Dance Theater Workshop.

More significantly, they have had an unmistakable influence on public policy. ACT UP's representatives have made serious inroads into the health establishment bureaucracy and become fixtures at most major scientific meetings and public hearings. At first, they thrust themselves uninvited and unwanted onto the dais. Later they earned grudging respect and bona fide speaking invitations.

But they have also won enemies.

ACT UP members are harsh toward those they deem enemies of the cause, and some say the organization plays dirty. In a typical display of theatrics, ACT UP shouted down then mayor Ed Koch at a gay history exhibit. Outraged by a scientific opinion with which they disagreed—and apparently fearful of losing attention for their cause—members splashed paint and pasted handbills on the house of Stephen C. Joseph, former New York City Health Commissioner, after he reduced estimates of the number of HIV-positive individuals from 400,000 to 200,000, based on more refined epidemiological data. When the organization decided that *New York Times* writer Gina Kolata was hostile to their initiatives for expanding access to new drugs, there was talk of decorating her shrubs with condoms or singing custom-tailored Christmas carols at her doorstep. Instead they settled on decals calling her the worst AIDS reporter in America, which were plastered on newspaper stands all over the city. John Leo, a columnist for *U.S. News and World Report,* was awakened by incessant telephone calls in the middle of the night after calling ACT UP a gangster group.

Probably their most pugnacious display came during high mass at St. Patrick's Cathedral. Some 5,000 protestors had gathered outside the Fifth Avenue landmark to castigate the Catholic Church's condemnation of homosexuality as a sin, its refusal to sanction the protective value of condoms because they are also a method of birth control, and its opposition to abortion and safe-sex education. Some demonstrators were dressed as bishops, others as clowns, and one man came in the habit of the Flying Nun. Several carried a huge mock condom tagged "Cardinal O'Condom." Inside the sacred building, protestors lay down in the aisles and chained themselves to the pews. Eventually the police came and hauled away on stretchers the demonstrators who refused to budge.

Then came the ignoble moment that has gone down in the annals of activist history. Tom Keane—Yale graduate, lapsed Catholic, and ACT UP member—accepted a communion wafer from Archbishop John Cardinal O'Connor, then crumbled it onto the floor, stating flatly, "Opposing safe-sex education is murder." Scandalized clergy rushed in to pick up the wafer pieces, the protestor was led away in handcuffs, and Cardinal O'Connor was photographed the next morning performing purification rites in the cathedral.

Despite the bad press it could sometimes generate, Martin Delaney turned to ACT UP when he learned that access to dextran sulfate had been choked off. He was convinced that Peter Staley was the man for the job.

Peter Staley did not have any formal training as an activist mastermind. With his short, curly hair and clean-shaven face, Staley looks younger than a man who recently turned thirty. But his deep brown eyes suggest the intensity that propelled him from a promising career as a Wall Street bond trader into the limelight as orchestrator of many of ACT UP's most dramatic direct actions.

Staley was raised on Philadelphia's exclusive Main Line. He attended Oberlin College, then defied its progressive traditions by joining Morgan Guaranty Trust and heading east to New York City's financial district. He was a Reagan supporter and a yuppie who led a straight-and-narrow life during working hours, then drifted uptown to drop in on the flourishing gay bar scene.

Until he learned that he was HIV-positive. As luck would have it, Staley was on his way to work one morning soon after hearing that grim news and stumbled across ACT UP's first demonstration. The organization had been founded just two weeks earlier, and the protestors were gathering to denounce the $10,000-a-year price tag on AZT and to focus attention more generally on government inaction on AIDS research. Demonstrators lay down in front of traffic on Wall and Broad streets, and the current FDA commissioner, Frank Young, was hung in effigy from the gallows in Trinity Church. Seventeen people were arrested. Staley was impressed with the fervor and commitment he saw, and made a beeline to an ACT UP meeting the next week. He has been an activist ever since.

Staley dresses casually, often in the popular ACT UP uniform—a black T-shirt decorated with the inverted pink triangle, and black jeans and boots. He talks softly about the sense of urgency that drives him. "We feel like we are in a bloody crisis," said Staley. "We think every minute counts. All we want is the same type of response that South Carolina got after the hurricane, what San Francisco got after the earthquake. But there is still no sense of emergency, still no leadership, still no one to hold accountable in the federal government."

Martin Delaney called Staley and explained that while many people believed dextran sulfate had antiviral properties, no one was able to get hold of the drug anymore.

Kowa had a branch office in Manhattan, and Staley agreed to organize a direct action against it. The event was meticulously orchestrated. On June 28, 1988, eleven people presented themselves to the receptionist at Kowa, pulled a long chain through the doorway, and handcuffed themselves to it. Startled, the receptionist jumped up from her desk and scurried to the safety of an inner office.

Mindful of the need for publicity, Staley had alerted Japanese television stations with correspondents in New York about the planned civil disobedience. But he grew concerned that the camera crews had not arranged a security clearance in advance, and in a bold display of chutzpah, Staley uncuffed himself from the chain of demonstrators and raced to the lobby to speak with security guards. Thinking fast on his feet, he told them, "I work with Kowa, and we're having a press conference. Please let the television crews in when they arrive."

Then he took the elevator back upstairs to Kowa's offices to join the others in handcuffs.

The police and the Japanese television crews arrived on the scene at almost the same time, and the lobby guards waved everyone through. Fortunately the cops were in good spirits that day, and no one was given a hard time. They even stopped hacksawing the chains of the demonstrators long enough to pose for the television cameras.

The story was big news in Japan that night. Shortly afterward, under activist prodding, the FDA wrote a letter to Japanese officials explicitly stating the agency did not oppose the sale of dextran sulfate to Americans. A compromise with Kowa was soon reached. Under the terms of the agreement, Americans were allowed to purchase dextran sulfate from three designated pharmacies in Japan, including one near the Tokyo airport. Stricter monitoring was imposed, however, with buyers required to sign a form indicating how many tablets they had purchased. Shipments of Japanese dextran sulfate once again flowed into the country, and Kowa never showed up in court to press trespassing charges against the demonstrators. Eventually all charges were dropped.

Meanwhile, the controversy swirling around dextran sulfate opened another Pandora's box: government import policies. With the sophisticated supply network starting up again, the FDA had its back to the wall in a most awkward way. Either it would have to continue to wink knowingly as thousands of dollars in unapproved drugs flowed into the country, or it would have to clamp down on desperate patients with no other alternatives.

While the agency considered its choices, the dextran sulfate bootleggers played a cat-and-mouse game with U.S. Customs. Most of the time, Customs officials waved through their shipments with no trouble, but periodically—and for no apparent reason—a packet of dextran sulfate was seized and turned over to the FDA. Project Inform's Martin Delaney would usually hear about the seizure and then call inside connections at the FDA to arrange for its release. Eventually the shipment was handed back, but usually patients first had to jump through the hoops of an elaborate bureaucracy.

"It makes no sense for you to detain the drug and then release it and put people through this agony time and time again," Delaney told Bill Schwemmer, a deputy commissioner in the FDA's Regulatory Affairs office. Apparently Schwemmer agreed, because a series of conference calls were held with top FDA officials, Martin Delaney, and New York activist/attorney Jay Lipner. Together they hashed out the terms of a new personal-use importation policy.

The announcement came at the annual National Lesbian and Gay Health Conference and AIDS Forum in Boston, scheduled shortly after Peter Staley and his friends occupied Kowa's offices. The week-long event, held in the summer of 1988, had already been lively. AIDS researchers at Harvard University were the targets of repeated jabs from ACT UP. Protestors dramatized their unhappiness with the pace of AIDS drug development by passing out cups filled with "Jim Jones Kool-Aid," to encourage comparisons with the Guyana massacre.

When FDA Commissioner Frank Young got up to speak, he was greeted with hisses; the FDA was perceived at the time, sometimes unfairly, as delaying access to promising drugs. Soon, though, the crowd stopped to listen—and many people were surprised to discover they liked what Young had to say. The hostility vanished and Young got a standing ovation.

Under the announced guidelines, individuals could import a three-month supply of most drugs if the product was purchased for personal consumption and not distributed commercially. The significant change from past practices was that importation by mail would be permitted, as long as the product's purpose was identified, no evidence of fraud or unreasonable risk could be uncovered, and purchasers signed letters saying the drugs were for their own use.

Although the guidelines were developed in response to interest in dextran sulfate, it was politically impossible to announce a liberal importation policy for only one drug. Frank Young's "Boston Bonanza" applied to all experimental drugs. Not everyone was euphoric about the decision. Some public health experts were shocked and talked about the return of the days when fraudulent and dangerous medication was widely available. There were even those who claimed the commissioner had gone mad.

In truth, Young had grown weary of hearing the FDA portrayed as a villain. After all, the agency had traditionally perceived itself as a benevolent overseer respected by the consumers it sought to protect. With the new importation policy, Frank Young hoped at last to win the affections of his critics. "How can I assure you that FDA is not doing business as usual in its fight against AIDS? And how can we work together better to defeat this dread disease?" he asked the audience. "I want you to know this disease is forcing us to reevaluate our procedures, refocus our priorities, and renew our public health commitment. . . . In fighting AIDS, FDA is committed to two important, but sometimes conflicting, principles—compassion and good science." It was the tension between those goals that sometimes put the FDA in a bind that left it vulnerable to criticism on all sides. The mixed reaction to the new import policy was a classic example of the no-win dilemmas the FDA sometimes faced.

There were other, more personal, motives for Young's announcement. In a comment made later that day to a reporter, he revealed a politician's concern for his own image. "There is such a degree of desperation and people are going to die. I'm not going to be the commissioner that robs them of hope," he said. Young also remarked that the FDA had a heart as well as a mind. With that, he had gone a bit too far, and one heckler responded by asking just what the FDA's mission really was—to provide the public with scientifically grounded consumer protection or with emotional support?

Despite its impact on public policy, dextran sulfate ultimately proved disappointing. Side effects often include diarrhea, slow-to-heal wounds, and minor liver toxicity, although most patients could tolerate these. More damning to the drug's prospects was the human body's inability to make much use of it. In October 1989, researchers at Johns Hopkins published the results of one small trial that found that less than 1 percent of dextran sulfate taken orally was absorbed into the bloodstream.

But the drug's medical value had never been the main issue in the debate over smuggling, buyers' clubs, or import policies. "It's not a question of whether dextran sulfate works," declared Martin Delaney. "It's a question of the right of people to do this. People with life-threatening illness have rights that supersede those of society to control their behavior."

That proclamation continues to be a rallying point for many in the activist movement.

8

THE PENTAMIDINE SAGA

❖

Concern for man himself and his fate must always
form the chief interest of all technical endeavors . . .
never forget this, in the midst of your diagrams and
equations.

—ALBERT EINSTEIN

EVERYONE INVOLVED WITH AIDS knew that *Pneumocystis carinii* pneumonia (PCP) was unmerciful. In the epidemic's early years some 80
percent of AIDS patients eventually developed the opportunistic infection; often it was the first clue of the lurking virus. Most patients
survived a first bout with the pneumonia. Many even survived a
second one. But each relapse was generally worse than the last,
leaving the lungs scarred with irreversible damage and breathing
increasingly labored. Few patients were able to withstand a third or
fourth battle with the tenacious infection. People with recurring PCP
eventually died a brutal death that has been likened to suffocation.

The horror of PCP was vividly described by Robert Mony, an
HIV-infected writer who recalled the painful and gruesome death of
a pneumonia-racked friend. "In his last days he had lost so much
weight that he looked like a concentration camp victim. He was too
weak to walk to the bathroom or take care of himself in any way."
The man refused to go back to the hospital, said Mony, preferring to
end his days at home, "soiling his bed, soaking the sheets with sweat

every night, frequently coughing up large gobbets of greenish phlegm."

Little wonder that Mony's own PCP diagnosis filled him with dread and foreboding. Little wonder that he pleaded with anyone who would listen to make prevention and treatment a priority.

More than most other AIDS-related conditions, PCP was also financially punishing. Hospitalization costs associated with a single acute episode ranged from $13,000 to $16,000, eating up a huge portion of the private and public health insurance dollars paying for AIDS care.

Both compassion and logic, then, clearly dictated that preventing pneumonia should have been a pressing public health priority. Instead, in what Michael Callen called "a scandal of unspeakable magnitude," PCP research fell by the wayside. Year after year, clinical investigators were unable to rise above the distracting disagreements that stymied their ability to design an appropriate trial. Pharmaceutical companies bickered about licensing rights. Resource shortfalls, a preference for studying the AIDS virus itself (which scientists found more alluring than studying specific infections), and leadership gaps also took their toll. It was business as usual in AIDS drug development.

But this time, while their leaders squabbled and delayed, AIDS patients and their allies swung into action.

COPING WITH A LETHAL PNEUMONIA

The drug that would create a new approach to AIDS drug research was named pentamidine. Developed in the early 1930s, initially to combat hypoglycemia, it had damaging side effects on the pancreas that forced researchers to set it aside. More than a decade later, the drug proved effective in preventing African sleeping sickness, and in the years after World War II, pentamidine was widely used overseas.

Long before AIDS, it had also been established that taking pentamidine by injection could halt the growth of *Pneumocystis carinii,* the organism that caused PCP, by impeding the synthesis of RNA and DNA. Pneumocystis is generally classified as a protozoan parasite, although recent studies indicate it may actually be a fungus. It was first isolated in Brazil in the early part of the twentieth century, where researchers found it in rats, and later it was seen in children living in orphanages, where malnutrition and overcrowding were often common.

Many completely healthy people are infected with *Pneumocystis carinii*, but the organism generally remains dormant and does no harm. Only when the body's immune system begins to weaken dramatically is the environment sufficiently hospitable for the pneumocystis to multiply. Small air sacs in the lungs known as alveoli can eventually become filled with the parasite, hindering an individual's ability to breathe. Fever and dry coughing also accompany infection. Occasionally the parasite will site itself outside the lungs, settling into the lymph nodes, bone marrow, spleen, or liver.

Only 100 cases of PCP had ever been documented in the medical literature until the 1960s. But soon the incidence began to inch steadily upward, spurred by the war against cancer, which relied heavily on immune-suppressing chemotherapy. The killer pneumonia was also seen in organ transplant patients, whose immune systems had been deliberately depressed to prevent organ rejection.

In 1974, Bactrim proved to be effective in treating the lethal pneumonia. Bactrim is a combination of two drugs—trimethroprim and sulfamethoxazole, hence the generic name trim-sulfa—and acts as a broad-spectrum antibiotic. Researchers eventually found that Bactrim could actually *prevent* PCP, and physicians began routinely administering it to patients at risk for the disease. Because it produced fewer adverse side effects, Bactrim soon replaced injectable pentamidine as the drug of choice. But patients who could not tolerate Bactrim or did not respond to it continued to get shots of pentamidine, and both drugs were the focus of scientific attention.

Incredibly, when the tidal wave of AIDS washed over the American landscape, twenty years of knowledge about PCP seemed to get swept away.

A handful of community physicians involved in AIDS had always been as interested in preventing PCP as in treating it. Joe Sonnabend, the heretical doctor who challenged the assumption that HIV was the sole cause of AIDS, had made PCP prophylaxis a standard of care since the early days of the epidemic by insisting that his patients take Bactrim. He could not enroll his patients in clinical trials; none were available back then. Nor were there skilled researchers on the scene to monitor them, which meant that potentially invaluable data about PCP prophylaxis was being scattered to the winds. Without rigorous scientific guidance, Sonnabend's efforts were dismissed as merely anecdotal. Yet his patients seldom got pneumonia.

Given the two decades of accumulated knowledge about PCP, a national AIDS czar might have insisted that preventing PCP be the bedrock of proper patient management and might have offered medical guidelines for providing it. But with no one in charge, local doctors resorted to educated guesswork and individual experimentation to determine dosage levels and the best way to have patients inhale the drug, so that the lungs could make optimal use of it. And even that was only for patients with access to state-of-the-art care—not poor people, not minorities, and not people in the nation's hinterlands.

Michael Callen discovered just how isolated many others were when he read that Ryan White had been hospitalized in Indiana with a bout of PCP. The young hemophiliac's courageous struggle against AIDS had made him America's poster boy and a household name. Yet when Callen tracked down his family, he discovered White's doctor knew nothing about PCP prophylaxis.

Callen proclaimed angrily, "If world-famous Ryan White did not know about the importance of PCP prophylaxis, there are undoubtedly thousands of Americans who are at this moment being denied what ought to be the standard of proper medical care for people at risk for AIDS."

Pentamidine was manufactured in Great Britain by May and Baker, a pharmaceutical firm that later became a subsidiary of the French company Rhone-Poulenc. The demand for pentamidine in the United States had been so slight that it was available only through the Centers for Disease Control, via its Parasitic Drug Service, which had been established to handle requests for drugs against rare tropical diseases. Pentamidine was flown from England to CDC headquarters in Atlanta, then shipped out to any physician who requested it on a compassionate-use basis. Until the early 1980s, those requests had been rare.

Then came a surge of calls for pentamidine, giving detectives at the Centers for Disease Control one of their earliest hints about an epidemic on the rise. At first the CDC kept up with the new requests. But as demand for pentamidine soared, the pressures on CDC staffers intensified. Illicit drug dealers weren't the only people sporting beepers in those days; CDC alert teams trafficking in pentamidine also began carrying the devices everywhere they went. Late-night telephone calls at home grew commonplace, with callers urgently announcing the arrival of a new shipment. Usually the hapless CDC staffer was then expected to race out to the airport to pick up the drug and speed it off to requesting physicians.

By the end of 1983 the CDC had received more than 2,200 requests for pentamidine. Morale plummeted as a result of the heavy and unexpected workload. Desperate to secure a more reliable supply of injectable pentamidine and ease the pressures on staff, the agency sought help from the National Organization for Rare Disorders, a patient advocacy group located in New Fairfield, Connecticut, and the New York–based Generic Pharmaceutical Manufacturers Association, the trade association for the generic drug industry. Together they tracked the world's remaining supply of pentamidine to a leaky warehouse in England. But the moment of hope when the drug was uncovered turned to dismay when the supply proved to be water-damaged and worthless.

Public health officials had just one alternative: to shop for an American company willing to fill the supply vacuum by manufacturing its own pentamidine. That shopping expedition proved to be a laborious one. The CDC had much the same experience as Sam Broder had when he was trying to involve drug companies in AIDS-related work. Most companies were still skeptical that marketing AIDS drugs would ever prove profitable.

After a string of refusals from pharmaceutical firms, the CDC finally interested an Illinois-based company named Lyphomed in the possibility of manufacturing injectable pentamidine. Lyphomed, founded by two physicians in 1969 to produce and sell generic drugs to hospitals, had earned its name by specializing in lyophilized products. Like instant coffee, a lyophilized drug is processed through freeze-drying in order to sustain its stability—after the drug is frozen, water is allowed to condense out and the drug is then packaged in dosage containers. Lyphomed's specialty was an important drawing card to the CDC since pentamidine was a lyophilized drug.

When the CDC first contacted Lyphomed in 1983, the company was owned by John Kapoor, a pharmacist from Bombay with an American doctorate in chemistry. Kapoor had signed on five years earlier, when Lyphomed was a troubled division of the Stone Container Corporation. In those days it was hemorrhaging money, showing monthly losses of $50,000 on sales that hovered around $1 million.

Over the next few years Kapoor was able to turn Lyphomed's fortunes around. By the time the company took center stage as the manufacturer of pentamidine in 1984, it was in such good financial shape that Kapoor actually saw the pentamidine deal as a potential tax write-off—not as the source for outrageous profits. Kapoor's wildest dreams could not have given him a hint that his first meeting with CDC officials would start him down the path toward becoming a millionaire one hundred times over.

At first Lyphomed and the CDC negotiated a straight contract deal in which the Feds would pay the company for each vial of injectable pentamidine it could produce. Lyphomed quickly churned out 3,000 vials.

As a carrot to the company, and to assure a steady supply of the drug, the FDA soon urged Lyphomed to take full responsibility for manufacturing and marketing pentamidine. It also advised the firm to apply for "orphan product" designation under the year-old Orphan Drug Act.

The Orphan Drug Act owes its existence in some measure to the dedication and determination of Abbey Meyers. As a mother of three children with Tourette syndrome, Meyers learned through wrenching personal experience how few drugs exist for most of the 5,000 rare diseases in the United States. In 1983 she helped found the National Organization for Rare Disorders as a clearinghouse of information and patient advocacy and has been fighting ever since to turn that situation around.

Sponsored by Congressman Henry Waxman, and guided through the shoals of the legislative process with Meyers's help, the Orphan Drug Act was signed into law by Ronald Reagan on January 4, 1983. The act originally defined a rare disease as one that occurs so infrequently that "there is no reasonable expectation that the cost of developing and making available in the United States a drug for such disease or condition will be recovered from sales in the United States."

Later, AIDS drugs proved that definition to be way off base.

The act created a lucrative incentive package to entice drug companies into rare-disease research. The crown jewel of the legislation is the seven-year exclusive right to sell an orphan product before other companies are allowed to compete on the marketplace. This helped stimulate research on new applications for drugs that had been developed long enough ago to be in the public domain and not protected under standard patent law, which is valid for only seventeen years. Until the Orphan Drug Act was passed, drug companies had little reason to become involved in research because competitors were able to sell identical products without restriction.

The Orphan Drug Act also provides research grants and tax credits that can reduce a company's tax obligations by about 70 percent, once they are combined with standard business deductions. The legislation has not made a huge dent in the treatment backlog for the 5,000 rare diseases, but it has helped. During its first nine years, sixty-nine orphan drugs were developed and approved for marketing.

Injectable pentamidine was the first AIDS drug to be approved under the Orphan Drug Act. Because no other American company owned the licensing rights, Lyphomed accepted the FDA's offer to pursue approval. The company was excused from conducting the usual clinical trials since previously published studies had long since demonstrated the drug's safety and effectiveness. Lyphomed's application for drug approval, written mainly by the CDC, was approved in just six months. In October 1984, Health Secretary Margaret Heckler announced the company had been granted the exclusive right to sell injectable pentamidine until 1991.

Those were heady days for the young firm. Later, as a swell of negative publicity bombarded Lyphomed, executives looked back to that era longingly. Windfall profits were all they could cling to as consolation.

The problem with the injectable variety of pentamidine was that it lodged primarily in the kidneys, adrenal glands, spleen, and liver; not enough of it got to the lungs, the major site of infection for AIDS patients. Nearly half of all patients who started on pentamidine had toxic reactions to it and had to change medications. Researchers badly wanted to find a more effective and safer way to administer the drug.

Although an aerosolized version of pentamidine had not been tried before in humans, the concept was appealing because it allowed a fine mist to be inhaled deeply into the lungs. One study showed that when rats were put into a room filled with aerosolized pentamidine, the drug penetrated their lungs in high concentrations while leaving other organs largely unaffected. Aerosolized pentamidine seemed to hold the greatest hope for preventing PCP altogether. Researchers in San Francisco and New York began to look for an effective nebulizer, a device that converts liquid pentamidine into an inhalable mist.

Everyone agreed it was only a matter of time before aerosolized pentamidine would be tested for human use. No one guessed almost five full years would elapse between the approval of injectable pentamidine and the day the FDA licensed the aerosolized drug.

Lyphomed had assumed its exclusive rights to produce and sell injectable pentamidine would automatically be broadened to include the aerosolized version. The FDA dispelled that assumption quickly and said that brand-new research had to be conducted. Lyphomed would have to compete with other manufacturers to win the new license.

Soon came another shocker. Lyphomed learned that Memorial Sloan-Kettering Cancer Center had entered into an agreement with Fisons, a billion-dollar pharmaceutical company based in Great Britain, to test aerosolized pentamidine and seek marketing approval. Lyphomed was especially enraged by the tactless timing of Fisons's announcement, which came the day after a Lyphomed-sponsored seminar on aerosolized pentamidine held at New York's Hilton Hotel on October 4, 1987. Assuming that no other manufacturer planned to conduct similar research, Lyphomed had used the occasion to go public with the details of its proposed study, revealing its enrollment targets, planned dosage, and the type of nebulizer it would use to aerosolize the drug. The following morning it was revealed that Donald Armstrong, who headed Sloan-Kettering's infectious disease division and who had chaired the Lyphomed seminar, was the principal investigator of the Fisons/Sloan-Kettering joint venture.

Lyphomed felt betrayed by the intrusion on its turf. Brian Tambi, who subsequently became president of Lyphomed, groused about Fisons's sudden interest in pentamidine. "A company that wasn't very much interested in the drug before suddenly wants to crowd us because they think there is money to be made," he said. Lawyers were consulted to develop grounds for a lawsuit against the pharmaceutical giant, but calmer heads prevailed. Lyphomed decided to take its aerosolized drug through the required testing process and concern itself with lawsuits only if it lost the race for approval.

Pneumopent, Fisons's version of aerosolized pentamidine, was designated an orphan drug first. Lyphomed was awarded the same status for its version, NebuPent, more than three months later.

While numerous firms can receive the initial orphan designation, only one actually wins the right to the seven-year marketing exclusive. The serendipitous applicant is the first one to meet all the FDA's requirements, which can be a somewhat arbitrary process not always related to the quality of the competing products or the date a firm actually submits its application. If one agency regulator has a bigger backlog or less training, or suffers a bout of ill health, the applications being reviewed are the likely losers.

For Fisons and Lyphomed, the race was on.

How the Government Bungled Its Trials

While the corporations were jockeying for position, the National Institute of Allergy and Infectious Diseases was in the process of bungling its own efforts to test aerosolized pentamidine. Its failure was a stunning indictment of the government's whole response to AIDS. Had the Feds been left to their own devices, aerosolized pentamidine would likely be an unlicensed drug to this day—and perhaps for years to come.

Part of the problem was that NIAID was struggling to get pentamidine trials off the ground while simultaneously working out the kinks of the government's first large AIDS clinical trial program. NIAID had won control of the research effort soon to be known as the AIDS Clinical Trial Group (ACTG), after jockeying for position with the National Cancer Institute in the mid-1980s.

NCI and NIAID, sister agencies of the National Institutes of Health, had both wanted to lead the government's AIDS research effort. Policymakers toyed briefly with the idea of having each institute pursue research independently, but scuttled the notion for fear of making the NIH look schizophrenic or inefficient.

There was logic enough for choosing the National Cancer Institute. Bruce Chabner, head of the Cancer Treatment Division at NCI, was particularly aggressive in his attempts to have NCI chosen for the job. NCI already had a well-established clinical trial system and the in-house expertise to run it. And two of its top scientists, Sam Broder and Bob Gallo, were AIDS research trailblazers.

But some officials at NIAID were pushing just as vigorously to head AIDS research. It made a certain amount of sense to put NIAID in charge, since AIDS is both an immune disorder and an infectious disease. Of course, NIAID's eagerness to dominate AIDS research reflected more than organizational logic—it also highlighted the thirst for the federal research dollars destined to flow to the lead agency. Not that anyone could have guessed the extraordinary amounts involved. No one imagined that by 1991, 47 percent of NIAID's $400-million annual budget would be devoted to AIDS.

Tony Fauci, who led the lobbying efforts on behalf of NIAID, began his career at the agency in 1968 after completing medical training at Cornell University. A combination of charisma, sharp intellect, and ambition helped him rise through the ranks of the bureaucracy. A specialist in immunology, he was initially hired as a clinical associate and moved on to various high-level administrative positions until being named agency director in 1984. Later he was given the additional title of director of the Office of AIDS Research at NIH. Fauci is also a brilliant researcher; in 1990, the *Science Citation Index* said that in the past decade his published writings were the eighth most frequently cited by other researchers, among the 1.3 million scientists who had been published around the world. He has his name on more than 725 scientific publications, including several textbooks.

In his spare time, Fauci indulged his predilection for racing cars and maintained an impressive record as a marathon runner, logging five to ten miles daily. About the only evidence that remained of his Brooklyn childhood was a strong accent, the basketball hoop he installed in his office so that he could shoot baskets to relieve stress, and lots of street smarts.

Backstage jockeying and political compromises determined how NIAID and NCI ultimately divided their AIDS research responsibilities, although the leadership at both agencies claim the disagreements never became serious. After informal negotiations, NIAID eventually earned the privilege—some would say it carried the burden—for conducting most of the work. NCI kept its hand in AIDS drug development, continuing to screen promising therapies and conducting basic virology research in its labs. Both Broder and Gallo remained closely involved. But NIAID was in charge.

Aerosolized pentamidine made it painfully obvious that the ACTG research program was bogged down. Pressure to get the drug tested in human beings had been mounting since injectable pentamidine had been approved. NIAID's own subcommittee said in February 1987 that this research ought to be a priority of the highest magnitude. Although some community physicians aerosolized the liquid drug for their patients, no patient was actually enrolled in a government-sponsored study until March 1988.

What happened in the intervening time offers an instructive glimpse into the federal bureaucracy and its interplay with scientists. It would have been a comic exercise in triviality were the consequences not so dire. As the months rolled by, numerous NIAID committees and subcommittees met to consider the best way to test aerosolized pentamidine. Lyphomed and Fisons proposed their own designs to government scientists, and so did other researchers. Each proposal in turn was rejected, revised, and resubmitted. Disagreements about which nebulizers to use, what size particles to spray into the lung's millions of tiny air sacs, and which drug dosage was most effective dominated the lengthy process.

In a particularly shortsighted move, government and academic researchers initially insisted on designing a placebo-controlled trial. But the window of opportunity for placebos had closed before trials ever got moving, because patients were unwilling to participate. One man explained why, and his thinking was straightforward: "I know aerosolized pentamidine works and I can get it through my doctors. Why should I join a study where I might be denied the drug?"

Here's what NIAID's protracted time line for testing aerosolized pentamidine actually looked like:

In April 1987, government officials contacted Lyphomed and suggested working together to develop an effective nebulizer to dispense aerosolized pentamidine. Lyphomed was noncommittal. After a few months of stalling, the company still would not say yes.

In May, Michael Callen and other AIDS activists met with Tony Fauci and begged him to issue interim guidelines urging physicians to provide prophylactic medicine—most likely pentamidine—to patients at high risk for PCP. Fauci refused. His reason: no data to support such an approach.

In June, East and West Coast academic researchers met in Washington, D.C., at the third International AIDS Conference, an annual event that brought together scientists, policymakers, drug companies, and patient advocates from around the world to discuss current developments in the epidemic. The investigators hoped to resolve their lingering differences about proper dosage and preferred delivery system so that trials could get moving at last. They failed to reach a consensus.

In August, a fifteen-person study conducted at San Francisco General Hospital, and described in *The Lancet*, lent more weight to the widely held conviction that aerosolized pentamidine was effective in treating PCP.

At about the same time a NIAID representative spoke with Fisons about its interest in aerosolized pentamidine. Fisons was open to collaboration. Further discussions took place the next month, with Fisons getting a detailed lecture on the structure and policies of the government trials system. Once again the studies failed to get off the ground because of all the technical disagreements.

In October 1987, Lyphomed and Fisons submitted competing study designs to NIAID. Each company proposed a very different delivery system and dosage. Important scientific claims were made for the rival studies, but government officials called them both flawed. An outside consultant, an expert in aerosol physics, was called in for an opinion.

In December, on the basis of the independent expert's report, NIAID scientists decided that perhaps both the Lyphomed and Fisons studies had scientific merit after all.

Still, negotiations dragged on. It was winter again, and for a moment the season of discontent seemed to be drawing to a close. Three trials, one for PCP treatment and two for prevention, finally appeared ready to move forward under a contract with Lyphomed.

In March 1988, one of the trials got started. But a few weeks later the FDA stepped in and requested changes in the study design of the other two. Another month was lost to further revisions.

NIAID did not actually begin to enroll patients in all three trials until June 1988. By then, community activists and their physicians were already a year into their own studies of aerosolized pentamidine.

When he held congressional hearings in April 1988, Ted Weiss was deeply discouraged with the federal government's response to AIDS. The FDA was under attack at the time, and so far as Weiss could tell, innovative thinking at NIAID was in equally short supply.

Tony Fauci was summoned to testify. Weiss intended to call Fauci to task for the lethargic pace at which NIAID was putting promising drugs into trials. Fauci tried to explain, pointing to staff shortages and the fact that his request to his superiors for 127 new employees had been answered with just 11 new slots. To push aerosolized pentamidine more rapidly through the system would have meant assigning one person the task as a full-time job, said Fauci. "Unfortunately, we just didn't have the staff to take someone and say, 'The only thing you're going to do for the next *x* number of months is aerosolized pentamidine.' . . . We couldn't afford to dedicate someone completely."

Weiss didn't think much of that response, and let Fauci know it. He reminded the AIDS research chief that his own committees had placed aerosolized pentamidine on the "highest priority" list. "You can understand how the people in the affected community, those who have the disease and who are struggling for their lives, feel when they hear that," Weiss said. "It just seems to me that we all ought to be up in arms and shouting from the rooftops that, in fact, we desperately need to have filled the resource request that you've made so they know, however these tests ultimately prove out, at least every effort is being made to undertake them."

It wasn't all Fauci's fault, of course. More than just extra staff would have been needed to guide pentamidine through the development process, even if NIAID had enough desks for new employees to sit at—which it did not. Someone over Fauci's head should have been greasing the wheels of the bureaucracy.

But extraordinary measures have never been Washington's response to the AIDS epidemic. The leaders all seemed to be asleep at the helm.

California congresswoman Nancy Pelosi pressed Fauci hard to show some empathy, urging him to think carefully about the perspective of people with AIDS. Just imagine, she said, that you live in San Francisco, that you have AIDS, and that you have had pneumonia once.

The tension mounted as Pelosi continued to develop her imaginary scenario. Suppose that you have heard from friends, and perhaps your own doctor, that aerosolized pentamidine seems to prevent pneumonia, she suggested. Then she said, "You know that many studies in San Francisco recommend it routinely and that it is available. You know that as of today, the delays in NIH trials is a problem that may not be solved this year. You know that your second or third bout of pneumonia will kill you." She then let fly a powerful question: "Would you take aerosolized pentamidine or would you wait for a study?"

As head of NIAID, and gatekeeper of the clinical trial system, Fauci clearly represented the establishment. That made his candor all the more stunning. Tony Fauci looked Nancy Pelosi straight in the eye and answered, "If I were in that situation and I had a bout of *Pneumocystis carinii* pneumonia, I would go for what is available on the street for me."

In one blunt statement, Tony Fauci had admitted that the system could not respond appropriately to the needs of people with AIDS, and virtually gave his blessing to the host of gray- and black-market activities exploding around the country.

9

LOOSENING THE
REGULATORY LEASH

❖

An element of abstract, or a divorce from reality,
entered into such calamities. Still, when abstraction
sets to killing you, you've got to get busy with it.

—ALBERT CAMUS,
The Plague

THE FOOD AND DRUG Administration knew that people with AIDS
were dangerously eager to experiment with unproven therapies and
it was determined not to lose all regulatory control. Motivated both
by compassion and realism, in the watershed month of March 1987,
FDA Commissioner Frank Young announced a new plan to release
promising but unapproved drugs.

The initiative had its roots in the FDA's long-standing compassionate-use tradition, but it was heralded as a dramatic shift in the
agency's regulatory procedures. Vice-President George Bush, who
chaired the Presidential Task Force on Regulatory Relief, and was
well known for his distaste for anything that might stifle corporate
profits, proclaimed that the FDA's regulatory leash had been loosened. The *Wall Street Journal* announced that "a giant step for the
sick and dying," ranking in significance with White House actions on
tax cuts and "Star Wars," had just been taken. A journalist for the

San Francisco Examiner said it marked the end of an era in which people with AIDS were "forced to visit clandestine clinics and foreign doctors."

While such unqualified enthusiasm soon waned, Young's initiative proved to have staying power.

TREATMENT IND

The proposal created a category of experimental drugs known as Treatment Investigational New Drugs (Treatment INDs). The initial concept allowed specially designated drugs for immediately life-threatening diseases to be sold after Phase I, under the condition that research continued; evidence also had to be presented to show that the drugs were not clearly ineffective or unreasonably dangerous, and that no other treatments were available.

Although this was far from a novel concept at the FDA—cancer drugs, for example, had long been made available to patients while still unapproved—there was a roar of reaction. During the forty-five-day period open for public comment, the FDA was flooded with more than 300 responses from almost every affected constituency.

The medical community was deeply divided. So were many of the AIDS advocacy groups. At the heart of the schism was the fact that the proposal did not require a drug to prove its effectiveness with certainty before being designated a Treatment IND. The critics charged that the door would be opened wide to fraud.

At hearings in April, veteran New York congressman Ted Weiss expressed the fear that Treatment IND could gut the FDA's power to regulate the drug industry. He also raised the haunting specter of another thalidomide disaster. Weiss's attitude toward expanding access to drugs is a curious illustration of the complexities that surround AIDS. His district includes the AIDS-devastated Greenwich Village community, and the liberal congressman had long been an ally of those fighting for more government dollars for AIDS research. Most of those allies also supported Treatment IND.

But Weiss had built a solid record of support for consumer protection and was better known for criticizing the FDA because it approved drugs too readily than for complaining when it didn't approve them swiftly enough. "The proliferation, in uncontrolled settings, of inadequately evaluated, potentially dangerous experimental drugs is a prescription for the premature deaths and needless suffering of large numbers of people," said Weiss at his hearing.

Weiss also suggested that the real motivation behind the Treatment IND program was to further the Reagan Administration's agenda to reduce government interference with private enterprise. His staff probed that point and managed to get hold of revealing internal documents from the Office of Management and Budget. A background paper showed that OMB wanted to eliminate the requirement to prove that benefits outweigh risks; to replace "the Commissioner may grant" with "the Commissioner shall grant" a Treatment IND; and to reverse the FDA's presumption against selling investigational drugs. Armed with these smoking guns, Weiss concluded, "OMB, under the guise of assisting people with AIDS, is, in fact, attempting to dismantle the whole regulatory process."

Around the time of the hearings, Jeff Levi, then executive director of the National Gay and Lesbian Task Force, also broke from the majority opinion in his community when he cautioned against using early results to justify distributing drugs. He used the example of suramin to make his point. That drug had been widely used to treat African sleeping sickness and, in the test tube, was able to prevent HIV from replicating, in a mode of action similar to AZT—by inhibiting the reverse transcriptase enzyme. In Phase I, the drug still seemed worth pursuing. In a September 1985 journal article published by Sam Broder and others at the National Cancer Institute, some side effects were acknowledged, including fever and urinary and liver abnormalities. The authors noted short-term improvements were disappointing but said, "The results provide a rationale for investigating longer-term regimens."

Tragically, during Phase II trials, involving forty-one gay men, more serious toxicities became apparent. Two patients died of liver failure while on the trial, and severe kidney and adrenal problems also surfaced. The authors, mostly academic researchers in California, said suramin should be abandoned. "Suramin is a toxic agent that shows no virologic, immunologic, or clinical benefit in patients with HIV-related disease," they wrote in March 1987. Levi shuddered to think of the likely death toll had the proponents of early access had their way and forced suramin to be handed out more freely.

Also in the camp of the doubters were such established institutions as the National Institutes of Health, the Mayo Clinic, and Johns Hopkins University, all of which questioned how Treatment IND would affect research. They asked why anyone would volunteer for clinical trials—and possibly get a placebo—if access to experimental drugs was possible through other means.

In an unusual twist of alliances, Martin Delaney of Project Inform organized a letter-writing campaign to thank Frank Young for proposing Treatment IND and another one to berate Jeff Levi for opposing it. To Levi activists wrote, "You are endangering our lives and giving the government an excuse to back away from the most responsive action they have ever taken on AIDS." The words were harsh and not entirely fair, but the activists were seldom known for their tact. The fevered debate continued.

FDA Commissioner Frank Young pushed hard for his original proposal. But five former commissioners expressed more concern, speaking with a single voice to demand that drugs give at least some indication that they worked before being sold, which had after all been the whole point of the hard-fought Kefauver Amendments. After considerable debate, the FDA adopted regulations on Treatment IND that stiffened efficacy requirements significantly. The phrasing was deliberately cautious, some said vague: a drug could be released for patient use if there was a "reasonable basis for concluding" that the product "may be effective." Full approval, by contrast, required much more certain proof that a drug worked. The FDA estimated that Treatment IND would get drugs to patients two to three years earlier than in the past.

The final rule, published in the *Federal Register* on May 22, 1987, and put into effect thirty days later, said drugs could be designated Treatment INDs if:

• The drug was intended to treat a serious or immediately life-threatening disease. ("Immediately life-threatening" was defined as a situation in which there was a "reasonable likelihood that death will occur within a matter of months or in which premature death is likely without early treatment.")

• No comparable or satisfactory alternative drug or other therapy was available to treat that stage of the disease in the intended patient population.

• The drug was currently under investigation in a controlled clinical trial or the trials have been completed.

• The sponsor of the controlled clinical trial was actively pursuing marketing approval with "due diligence."

Despite the brouhaha it engendered, the Treatment IND proposal essentially codified vague but long-established compassionate-use practices. The new regulations, wrote two Columbia University professors, were clearly not "the lead paragraph in the obituary of the FDA."

THE PECULIAR LIMITS ON TRIMETREXATE

On February 16, 1988, almost a year after the Treatment IND regulations had been released, trimetrexate, used to treat PCP, which is still the leading killer of people with AIDS, became the first AIDS drug to be awarded Treatment IND status. When he announced the designation, Young said it reaffirmed the "FDA's commitment to broaden early patient access to promising experimental treatments for AIDS."

But his announcement about trimetrexate had a disturbing flaw. To qualify for the drug, a patient was required first to have an adverse reaction to the two drugs that had already been approved for the treatment of PCP, namely injectable pentamidine and Bactrim.

Some patients suffering from pneumonia did not respond to either of those medications, but had no adverse reactions to them, either; the drugs were merely ineffective. By a logic not wholly comprehensible, those patients could not get trimetrexate under the terms of the Treatment IND. "This not only defies common sense, it is contrary to the aim of the regulations," said David Barr, then an attorney with Lambda Legal Defense and Education Fund, an advocacy group that uses test-case litigation to protect the rights of gay citizens.

In making its stick-with-the-status-quo decision, FDA regulators had ignored the wishes of patients, the advice of physicians, and the recommendation of the National Institute of Allergy and Infectious Diseases.

*   *   *

The guidelines for the trimetrexate Treatment IND were designed principally by Ellen Cooper, the FDA regulator who had earlier won so much praise for rushing AZT through the approval process. Critics said she must have been wearing her black hat at the time, because her hard-line approach to trimetrexate infuriated many activists. Martin Delaney called her "rigid and adamant in her belief" and said she had failed to consider how her medical decisions affected people's lives.

A kinder perspective held that Cooper initially made by-the-book scientific decisions and did not approach AIDS with sufficient flexibility. The narrow eligibility criteria established for trimetrexate also reflected the FDA's reluctance to apply the Treatment IND designation too liberally. Although Commissioner Frank Young clearly favored the innovation, it apparently was making some of his top regulatory experts uncomfortable.

The fracture within the agency was illustrated in one angry confrontation between Martin Delaney and Ellen Cooper. During the heated exchange over Treatment IND, Cooper said, according to Delaney, "If this community thinks that it's going to get much earlier access to drugs under these regulations, it's fooling itself."

Delaney countered, "But that's exactly what your commissioner has said all over the airwaves repeatedly, that a major change has taken place."

Cooper paused a moment before responding, "Well, then, I think he has raised some false hopes there."

In an interview years later, Cooper denied opposing the Treatment IND process arguing that the real issue was the dearth of effective drugs. Hopes that Treatment IND would release a backlog of drugs were unrealistic, said Cooper, because few promising AIDS therapies had emerged from the testing pipeline to offer a glimmer of hope.

One big problem with Treatment IND was that pharmaceutical companies were reluctant to apply for the special designation, partly because of liability concerns. Although patients who were prescribed drugs on Treatment IND had to give informed consent, the company seldom had a voice in designing the forms in use, and thus felt vulnerable to litigation. Some doctors also refused to prescribe Treatment IND drugs partly because of the paperwork involved and partly because of their own fears about liability. Paula Sparti, a Florida physician with a large AIDS practice, conceded that such indifference from the medical community might sound extraordinary but insisted it was real. "I know it is unbelievable, almost unfathomable, that they can go to sleep at night based on that, but I hear that every day," she said.

Also, the way that Treatment IND status would affect a company's drug application was ill-defined. There was talk that the FDA should prod companies into the program by agreeing to speed the final review and approval process in exchange for applying for Treatment IND status, but no such action was ever taken.

One of the most controversial elements of Treatment IND was that it permitted companies to charge for still unapproved drugs, although theoretically only enough to recoup their costs. The ruling permitted companies to "sell but not commercialize" experimental medications, a major change from the free distribution required in the past, when promising drugs had been made available on a compassionate-use basis. Allowing drug companies to recover their costs was probably the only way to entice firms into the Treatment IND program, but critics said it might create a financial bonanza for the pharmaceutical companies. Safeguards to discourage profiteering were built into the system, but they were flaccid. A further problem was that most insurance policies refused to pay for experimental medications, so Treatment IND drugs would likely be available only to people with ample resources.

But the biggest drawback to Treatment IND had nothing to do with cost. Rather, it was the vague criteria used for granting Treatment INDs. There remained a nagging question. What did the FDA really mean when it said drug companies could apply for Treatment INDs after proving that their products "may be effective"?

Jay Lipner tried to find out. Lipner was diagnosed with AIDS in March 1987, the month he had his first bout of pneumonia, and he died 4½ years later, in November 1991. In the years that he battled illness, Lipner also became a shrewd and influential strategist. His first move was to turn over the reins of his lucrative law practice to his partner in order to volunteer at Gay Men's Health Crisis, where he helped AIDS patients file for government entitlement benefits. Soon he was making a name for himself as a behind-the-scenes force to be reckoned with at the FDA.

The Texas-bred attorney spent much of the 1970s working as an antipoverty lawyer with a public-interest law firm in Washington. In 1979 he came to New York City to press Attorney General Robert Abrams's lawsuit against the polluters of Love Canal—a position that introduced him to key players in the state Health Department. Those connections, coupled with his knowledge of Washington rule-making, served him well. "I'm reasonable, I know what I'm talking about, and I won't go away," said Lipner in explaining his influence.

The young attorney was often on the scene when activists were trying to pin down the FDA about its Treatment IND regulations and guidelines. He recalled the frustration of those sessions. "I asked the same question over and over again until I was blue in the face. . . . What does 'may be effective' mean? If it is not the same thing as 'is effective,' if it is not the same standard as a new drug application, what is it? I still do not have the answer to the question," said Lipner with evident consternation.

In effect, Treatment IND was initially treated only as a bridge between the end of formal drug testing and the official stamp of marketing approval. That's not what patients had in mind; they cared less whether trials definitely showed that a drug worked than about finding out for themselves as soon as possible. Critics began complaining that all the restrictions on Treatment IND had gutted the program. Hostility toward the FDA flared at congressional hearings called by Ted Weiss in April 1988. The trimetrexate issue was on the front burner.

Despite his earlier reservations about Treatment IND, Weiss was angry at the niggling distinction between patients who were intolerant to other drugs and those who did not respond. He asked, "Why is trimetrexate being limited to persons who have severe or life-threatening reactions to both standard therapies for PCP—and not given to others who do not respond to the standard drugs, when failure to respond is tantamount to death? The distinction escapes me."

Barry Gingell also expressed his distress. Gingell, a New York physician, was director of medical information for Gay Men's Health

Crisis until his death from AIDS. Gingell angrily told listeners at the Weiss hearings that the Treatment IND program appeared to be "smoke and mirrors."

Another eloquent voice of protest was that of Jim Eigo. Eigo's ascetic manner and detached air have earned him the nickname of ACT UP's St. Francis of Assisi. He is pale and muscular, his hair worn back in a ponytail. At the sometimes volatile meetings of activists, he is soft-spoken, the man who tries to be a peacemaker.

There was little in Eigo's past to prepare him for his role as an outspoken political player or a scientific expert. A graduate of the California Institute of the Arts, he has been in New York since the 1970s, when he arrived with the ambition of publishing his own fiction. But for many years, Eigo set his art aside to devote most of his waking hours to the cause of AIDS activism. His tiny, rent-stabilized studio apartment in the East Village—a neighborhood where drug use is the leading cause of AIDS—served as his office.

Although he is HIV-negative, Eigo said it was the force of circumstances, the direct experience of tragedy that propelled him into action. "I live on Avenue A, I am a playwright, and I am a gay man," said Eigo. "And so in these past few years, I have seen my neighborhood, my profession, and my kind devastated."

During the debate over Treatment IND, Eigo spoke up often. He sounded deeply disappointed when he described the failure to get more drugs designated as Treatment INDs and complained about "a tragic narrowing of a program that once promised so much." He also reminded policymakers that people cannot "ethically be asked to wait for a drug until all the bureaucratic niceties have been fulfilled when their only alternative is death or grave deterioration in quality of life."

Martin Delaney also spoke out in protest. After months of watching hopefully, he said he had been forced to conclude that Treatment IND was "little more than a public relations exercise which holds little or no promise for improved access to treatment."

Commissioner Frank Young tried to allay the distress. At the Weiss hearings, he listened to Jay Lipner's complaints, then handed Lipner his business card and asked him to come to Washington for a meeting.

Lipner and David Barr from Lambda flew down to the capital shortly afterward.

As Lipner told the story, Young was flanked by Ellen Cooper and a number of other top FDA officials. Lipner opened the meeting with his familiar complaint, saying the FDA had not implemented its Treatment IND regulations properly. Again, he tried to pin down a definition of the controversial phrasing "may be effective."

"What is the standard that the FDA is going to apply to Treatment INDs if it's not the gold standard needed for approval?" Lipner demanded.

Officials said the appropriateness of the Treatment IND designation was determined on a case-by-case basis, adding that policies for particular drugs could not be revealed because the information was proprietary.

"Okay, are there in fact any drugs that meet the standard, whatever it is?" Lipner asked at the meeting.

Although the answer was no, officials added that they were expecting to use the designation soon. Jay Lipner and David Barr were not terribly reassured by that pledge, but it seemed impossible to push the agency any further just then. Determined to gain some advantage from a private meeting at which the commissioner was eager to please, they switched subjects and raised their concerns about the restrictive trimetrexate Treatment IND. In the process they got an inside look at just how shaky Frank Young's grip on his own agency had become.

Lipner remembered Young saying physicians could request trimetrexate for their patients on a compassionate-use basis if they didn't qualify for the Treatment IND.

According to Lipner, Cooper and her boss, James Bilstad, spoke up to contradict Young point-blank. "They interrupted to say, 'No, we don't like that. We don't like compassionate use because it will interfere with research,'" Lipner recalled.

"Wait a minute," Lipner said to Young's underlings. "You've got the commissioner of the FDA sitting here on my left, telling me the solution to the problem is to make a compassionate-use request. And you're telling me that you don't like that solution. Would you please tell me who is right?"

Lipner never got a direct answer to his question. Instead the chief

FDA counsel spoke up to complain about his aggressive bluntness, and said he had no right to barge in and demand answers.

"I felt it fairly extraordinary for the head of a major agency to be contradicted by his staff in front of two outsiders," said Lipner. "It was quite open."

Although Lipner and Barr got little satisfaction that day, they continued the public wrangling and behind-the-scenes arm-twisting to gain wider release of trimetrexate. Lambda eventually threatened to bring a lawsuit if the drug was not given to patients who failed to thrive on other drugs.

Finally the FDA came around. Several months after the Weiss hearings in April, the agency broadened the terms of its Treatment IND, making trimetrexate available to anyone who did not respond to injectable pentamidine or Bactrim.

Later, Cooper, like other Monday-morning quarterbacks at the FDA, admitted that in the absence of any other effective treatment options, trimetrexate should have been more accessible from the outset. "In retrospect, would we have done it differently, would we have acted faster?" Cooper asked rhetorically in an interview. She answered her own question with one word: "Yes."

Despite the trimetrexate concession, the frustration over Treatment IND continued to grow. One of the most telling blows came when the Presidential Commission on the HIV Epidemic issued its final report in June 1988 and declared unreservedly that the expanded access program was "not meeting the needs of persons with AIDS or advanced HIV-related illness."

ACT UP was convinced that for either bureaucratic or philosophical reasons, the FDA was still delaying access to drugs. By the summer of 1988, the momentum for change quickened. "It became increasingly clear to the scientific and political communities that whatever the FDA was doing, it was doing wrong. It was not moving fast enough, it was not setting the right priorities," said Jay Lipner.

"The priorities should be to save lives. The priorities should be to help people who have diseases for which there are no treatments. There has to be some risk taken."

Risk-takers within the federal bureaucracy seemed to be in short supply.

o   o   o

On October 11, 1988, ACT UP vented its frustration. In a demonstration conceived by David Barr, more than 1,000 protestors converged in Rockville, Maryland, and virtually shut down operations at FDA headquarters. Eighteen months after its birth, ACT UP had earned a reputation for being audacious, theatrical, and shrewd and it showed all three of those characteristics that fall day. As police dressed in full riot gear moved forward, demonstrators chanted, "Shame, shame, shame," and "Arrest Frank Young." Many lay still on the ground, holding up placards reading: "Rest in Peace. Killed by the FDA" and "I Died on Placebo." There were 176 arrests made, mostly for loitering, and the story got headlines across the nation.

Eight days after the ACT UP demonstration, and, not so coincidentally, three weeks before the 1988 presidential election, the FDA announced new regulations to speed drug approval. This time, said Frank Young, the agency would formally codify the ad hoc steps taken the year before to speed AZT through the testing pipeline.

The regulations, referred to as Sub-Part E, encouraged sponsors to consult early with the FDA. In the past, a firm often ran a drug through its paces, then brought the data to the FDA, only to be told it was flawed and that parts of the studies would have to be redone. By becoming involved sooner, the FDA hoped to nail down a trial design that would work before too much time was lost. The new approach also expanded Phase II trials so that more safety and efficacy data could be collected more swiftly. The idea was to bypass the last set of trials altogether in the case of drugs for life-threatening diseases. Finally, the regulations stated that in certain unusual situations the FDA was prepared to do some of its own research if the sponsor was unable to provide adequate data on a promising drug.

Many activists called the Sub-Part E regulations mere window dressing because pharmaceutical companies were not required to consult early with the FDA. The National Gay and Lesbian Task Force criticized the FDA's announcement as a "pre-election gambit rather than a serious attempt to make promising experimental therapies available." ACT UP New York made the same point a bit more colorfully, claiming in its *FDA Action Handbook,* an internal background piece on the agency, that "the 1988 Republican campaign wants to have an AIDS feather in its rather tattered cap."

But the activists scoffed too quickly. Despite continued dissatisfaction with some of the specific uses of Treatment IND, that initiative, coupled with the Sub-Part E regulations, gradually began to recast the way in which the drug companies and the FDA conducted their business. Over the next few years, the FDA showed an increasing willingness to take more chances in its application of Treatment IND. Jarred by criticism from its many constituencies, the agency gradually began to rethink its own philosophy. The evolutionary shift was most apparent as the once sacred notion that the FDA's sole mission was to *protect* the public health gave way to a growing consensus that it was also in business to *enhance* the public health. And that meant getting safe and effective drugs to the American public as quickly as possible.

10

GRASSROOTS TRIALS COME OF AGE

Activists Seizing Control

A physician is obligated to consider more than a diseased organization, more even than the whole man—he must view the man in his world.

—HARVEY CUSHING

WHILE THE FEDERAL GOVERNMENT tinkered with the issues of Treatment IND and clinical trial design, and while Lyphomed and Fisons were locking horns in the battle for exclusive marketing rights to aerosolized pentamidine, activists and their physicians seized control.

One of the extraordinary accomplishments of the community forces galvanized against AIDS was the ability to provide data scientifically rigorous enough to permit the FDA to approve aerosolized pentamidine. The clinical trials engineered in the gay communities of New York and San Francisco ushered in a radical change in the way drugs are tested in this country.

The Community Research Initiative and the County Community Consortium

Mathilde Krim, Joseph Sonnabend, Thomas Hannan, and Michael Callen first met in a small Greenwich Village church on West 11th Street in 1984, not realizing they were going to map uncharted land. Their first meetings were mainly about bottlenecks in the drug development process and what could be done to ease them.

But over the next three years they began to lay the groundwork for community-based research. The concept is to test drugs in the cities and neighborhoods where people with AIDS actually live, rather than in a more removed academic medical setting. Doctors on the frontline of the epidemic, known and trusted by their patients, generally administer the experimental medications. Although there is a tradition of community trials in cancer research, they are run by the National Cancer Institute and have never included significant input from patients themselves. AIDS research innovators took a very different tack.

A special virtue of grassroots studies is that they empower local physicians. Because they have taken the painful journey from diagnosis to death with hundreds, sometimes thousands, of AIDS patients, these doctors have the sense of urgency that comes with firsthand experience. They also know the frustrations of bearing witness on a daily basis to the consequences of disfiguring fungal diseases, sight-stealing cytomegalovirus, and other numerous infections they cannot cure. "Traditional researchers thought that community doctors would not be sophisticated enough to run trials. But actually they were highly sophisticated," said Mathilde Krim, who helped lay the groundwork for the historic innovation. "After all, they had been managing the disease for years."

At first, community-based research was a measure of desperation, a reflection of deep dissatisfaction with the government's approach to clinical trials. "The current system has not produced the goods . . . the emperor has no clothes," said Nathaniel Pier, an activist and doctor who died of AIDS in 1988.

In its early days, the innovative concept attracted more ridicule than respect from the scientific establishment. "They sneered," Krim recalled. "But we paid no attention."

Skeptics said it would be impossible to take into account all the variables that arise in a community setting, and that might affect results—in particular, they were concerned that enrollment would be almost unrestricted. Some added that the typical primary-care physician was untrained in the laborious process of collecting and evaluating data on new drugs, and that doctors with busy private practices didn't have time to complete the necessary paperwork and didn't understand why it had to be done. The critics droned on relentlessly with a single theme: that the scientific integrity of drug trials was going to be compromised.

But the community-based research advocates stuck to their guns. "This community is not prepared to roll over and die," declared Thomas Hannan, a New York–based activist, sounding the charge that forced activists to take matters into their own hands. Gradually the harsh opposition subsided.

Joe Sonnabend helped plant the seeds for the idea by informally collecting data on patients experimenting with unapproved drugs. One of his first research projects was isoprinosine, a drug approved in dozens of countries around the world but left in regulatory limbo here. Although isoprinosine had helped give rise to the Mexican connection and launched the AIDS underground, at first no one was collecting data on patients who were using it.

Although Sonnabend's suspicion that isoprinosine might help rebuild ravaged immune systems was not borne out at the time, his work showed that researchers could tap into the wealth of information being generated in doctor's offices. Ironically, the *New England Journal of Medicine* published a provocative study many years later indicating that Sonnabend's suspicions may actually have been right—isoprinosine did appear to slow the progression of AIDS.

But at the time, his chief contribution was in paving the way for the birth of the Community Research Initiative (CRI).

CRI opened for business in 1987. Although it was shut down four years later by financial and managerial setbacks, it had by then earned an important slot in the annals of AIDS research history. "We take our direction from the community's needs," said Bernard Bihari, who served first as CRI's medical director and later as executive director. "They tell us what problems they want to solve. We won't do a study unless it is going to be attractive to people with AIDS."

At CRI, proposals were developed by knowledgeable individuals—physicians, patients, and ethicists with strong ties to the AIDS community—a startling reversal of the usual pattern. Two full-time physicians carried out almost all the research on three floors of the aging West 26th Street building in Manhattan's Chelsea neighborhood that it shared with the PWA Health Group. Although that setup was a big improvement from the days when CRI squatted in the back of recreation rooms at the Gay Men's Health Crisis offices, the facilities were never plush; researchers often sat in stairwells to interview patients, and piles of paperwork were stacked everywhere in overcrowded rooms.

CRI's centralized approach to community-based research stood in curious contrast to San Francisco's County Community Consortium (CCC), where research is conducted at doctor's offices throughout the Bay Area.

CCC was the brainchild of Don Abrams and Paul Volberding, two very different, sometimes very competitive men, each a major player on the AIDS research scene. Although their offices sit side by side at San Francisco General, the city's only municipal hospital, each has carved out his own territory.

Paul Volberding was the principal investigator on the pathbreaking Protocol 019 study, which showed the value of intervening in the course of HIV infection by using AZT before symptoms appear. He is a big player in the AIDS Clinical Trial Group system, NIAID's research network, and very much a part of the medical establishment. Good looking and charismatic, Volberding has also been something of a media darling. Raised on a dairy farm in the Midwest, he trained at universities in Minnesota and Utah before making his way west to San Francisco as chief of oncology at San Francisco General Hospital. On Volberding's first day of work, a colleague introduced him to a patient with Kaposi's sarcoma, and he has stayed at the forefront of AIDS research ever since.

Don Abrams made his reputation as a central figure in community-based research. Although firmly planted in the scientific camp—he has been criticized by some AIDS activists as being too rigid and traditional—Abrams's efforts to develop a new approach to AIDS drug testing also made him a frontiersman.

The genesis of the County Community Consortium was a series of lively meetings designed to improve communication between academic and community physicians. These groups had long been at odds because their agendas were so different; the academics took a traditional approach to science while the community doctors were more focused on getting the latest therapies to their desperate patients. Under the rubric of CCC, which got its formal start in March 1985, two years before CRI, they managed to set aside many of these differences for a common goal: finding drugs that worked.

Unlike CRI, the County Consortium kept decision-making authority in the hands of physicians, not patients. Don Abrams resented efforts by patient advocates to wrest authority for establishing research priorities from the hands of scientists, and feared the consequences of such actions. "It should be the scientists and the investigators who say what should be studied," he insisted.

Despite differing approaches, the County Community Consortium and the Community Research Initiative were both historic departures from traditional research models. Their work—indeed, their very existence—had an impact that reverberates through the medical establishment to this day.

TESTING PENTAMIDINE IN LOCAL SETTINGS

For its first public appearance, CCC chose to study the long-delayed aerosolized pentamidine. An early attempt to get research off the ground had to be scuttled when Burroughs Wellcome and the National Cancer Institute launched the AZT trials. Initially, patients testing AZT were not permitted to use pentamidine; the prospect of being excluded from AZT studies, which were generating so much enthusiasm, discouraged most patients from enrolling in the pentamidine trial.

When the Phase II AZT trial was halted in September 1986, Don Abrams and the CCC again geared up to test pentamidine. Feelers were sent out to NIAID asking whether the agency would fund such a study if it were based in the offices of local doctors, rather than in a more traditional research setting. Tentative word came back that the application was likely to fly.

Don Abrams and Gifford Leoung, who became the study's principal investigator, worked on the study design together. Their first big decision: no placebos would be used.

That decision was in part traceable to an inglorious Bactrim study launched three years earlier by Margaret Fischl, an academic researcher who was also involved in pivotal AZT studies. Fischl's trial was designed to study whether Bactrim could prevent *Pneumocystis carinii* pneumonia in AIDS patients. Half of her patients got the drug; the rest received no treatment at all.

Fischl defended the placebo controls, which were approved by an ethical review committee, claiming there was no proof that Bactrim would work in AIDS patients. And that was true. But more significant was that a body of medical literature had already proven that Bactrim prevented PCP in patients with other immune deficiencies. Fischl knew about those studies. In fact, she mentioned them when she published the results of her own research. She also knew that even without formal proof, Bactrim was being widely prescribed to people with AIDS. But, like so many other mainstream researchers, Fischl had been schooled in mainstream ideas, which had placebos as their foundation, and she was not prepared to change her mind, even in the face of a life-threatening new disease. She refused to alter her trial design.

The Bactrim debacle was well known to Abrams and the patient community in San Francisco. It had made them furious. Determined to avoid the much-criticized placebo, Abrams and Leoung divided their patients at random into two groups receiving low doses of aerosolized pentamidine—either 30 or 150 milligrams twice a month—and one group getting a higher dose, 300 milligrams once a month. Eligible candidates had to have either survived one bout of pneumonia or been diagnosed with Kaposi's sarcoma or some other AIDS-related condition. They were barred from having used another drug known to be effective against PCP, but were permitted to continue on AZT.

A few months after NIAID's subcommittee called aerosolized pentamidine a high-priority drug, the FDA approved Don Abrams's three-arm study. Then NIAID delivered a crushing blow that almost derailed the whole concept of community research. Despite its earlier expression of interest in the local study, officials turned down CCC's request for funds. Insiders told Abrams that NIAID bureaucrats still considered grassroots research too novel. In light of its own failure to move pentamidine into trials, supporting the San Francisco effort would have been a mark of courage. NIAID did not have the vision to do so.

"We were left truly stranded," said Abrams. Undaunted, he and Leung went hustling for other subsidies and managed to find them. The University of California stepped into the breach with $50,000 in stopgap funds, and Lyphomed later provided additional capital.

Enrollment in the Consortium's landmark study moved swiftly. Within four months, 408 patients, under the care of seventy-three different physicians, had signed up. The study continued for eighteen months.

Meanwhile, New York's Community Research Initiative launched its own aerosolized pentamidine trial. The final push at CRI had come after a disappointing May 1987 meeting with Tony Fauci, an infamous session at which Michael Callen and others had pleaded for federal guidelines advising doctors nationwide to use pentamidine to prevent PCP. Fauci had refused. Callen was intensely disillusioned. When he flew back to New York from Washington, he told colleagues, "We're going to have to test it ourselves."

CRI never applied for official FDA authorization, but its trial was patterned on the CCC experiment already under way in San Francisco. Lyphomed came up with hundreds of thousands of dollars to subsidize the CRI trial and ninety physicians agreed to participate. More than 200 patients were soon enrolled.

Together, the New York and San Francisco trials made history.

On May 1, 1989, Lyphomed brought its aerosolized pentamidine trial data before an FDA advisory committee; the documentation was based largely on data reported by the County Community Consortium trial, and CRI provided backup information, especially about toxicity. It was going to be a make-or-break test for community-based research.

Lyphomed had earlier received the FDA's permission to distribute aerosolized pentamidine on physician request through the Treatment IND program. Now formal approval was within reach. It looked as though Lyphomed was going to beat Fisons to the finish line, and an infamous chapter of AIDS drug development might finally draw to a close.

But many people feared the FDA committee would not consider the data good enough. In her introductory remarks, Ellen Cooper pointed out that CCC's study entailed less-stringent-than-usual monitoring and record keeping, adding as a note of reassurance that FDA auditors who had visited the site of the San Francisco trial had no cause to question the data's basic reliability.

Top CCC investigators presented their statistical analyses and other study data in great depth. They even revealed a few glitches: ten participants had been "so enthusiastic about the trial that they enrolled twice," admitted David Feigal, a researcher who, ironically, succeeded Cooper as FDA's antivirals division head several years later. That quirk, he assured reviewers, had later been corrected.

CRI representatives then staged their own presentation, designed in part to convince the FDA they took scientific research principles seriously. Robert Mony brought a human face to the proceedings as he explained how access to aerosolized pentamidine had meant the difference between his life and death.

Eighteen months earlier, Mony had been diagnosed with pneumonia. During his painful ten-day hospitalization, a tube was inserted through his side to keep his lung inflated while he was given Bactrim intravenously—until he developed an allergic reaction to it. Mony was eventually declared free of infection, but he lived with the terror that the pneumonia might return. Given his allergies, there was little else that could have been done for him. When the CRI trial was developed, he signed up eagerly. Mony told the committee the trial's biggest enticement was the fact that it was set up by people with firsthand experience of AIDS: "I knew that it would be conducted with my best interests in mind and that I would be surrounded by sympathetic, nonjudgmental people and that I would not be treated as a guinea pig and allowed to get sick again and perhaps die, just to accumulate yet more data on untreated AIDS."

Michael Callen was one of the last speakers to appear at the day's session. As he talked about friends he had lost to AIDS, Callen painted a vivid picture of PCP's brutality. "I have witnessed firsthand the tremendous, unnecessary suffering caused by PCP—people with AIDS grasping for breath, twitching on respirators, unable to speak."

Then he spoke with all the passion of an AIDS survivor about the urgent need for effective PCP prophylaxis—and the disastrous consequences of the government's failure to spread that word. "No one in the AIDS establishment seemed to have any interest in the clinical observations of the physicians on the frontlines of this epidemic," he said. "Frustrated, the AIDS community has been forced to roll up its sleeves and do the research necessary to prove to the satisfaction of the AIDS establishment what community physicians and many people with AIDS have known for some time, that prophylaxis saves lives. . . . The AIDS community has done an end run around Federal incompetence and indifference."

CCC and CRI both put on persuasive performances. At the end of the day, the FDA committee voted unanimously to approve aerosolized pentamidine for the prevention of *Pneumocystis carinii* pneumonia. Full agency approval came six weeks later, on June 15, 1989, a little more than two years after AZT. Lyphomed was granted the exclusive right to market aerosolized pentamidine for PCP prophylaxis until June 15, 1996. That assured not only the drug's widespread availability but reimbursement through most public and private insurance policies. At the same time, the National Institutes of Health finally issued guidelines urging physicians to provide prophylactic treatment against PCP to susceptible patients.

For the first time in modern history, the lifeline of a new drug had been extended to patients solely on the basis of data gathered in a community setting.

AN INNOVATION GOES MAINSTREAM

On the heels of the stunning pentamidine success, interest in community-based research built steadily. The bold experiment had already gotten a big boost when the Presidential Commission on the HIV Epidemic said in its final report that the failure to involve community-based physicians in research was "an underutilization of valuable resources." CRI was specifically mentioned as an effective model, and the commission urged that federal funds be made available for other such grassroots research programs.

In the fall of 1988, Congress moved on that recommendation, funding a $6-million pilot program to seed community-based clinical trial programs around the country. For the first time ever, federal funds became available to test AIDS therapies beyond the walls of the National Institutes of Health and the ACTG sites, which were located mostly at universities and medical centers.

NIAID was put in charge, and the agency soon issued a request for proposals. Within a month, NIAID was flooded with calls from would-be local researchers asking how to apply for funds. Eventually, more than 700 application requests poured in. Sixty-six community-based health organizations actually completed the 193-page application by the due date.

It was the largest number of proposals ever received by NIAID for a single contract solicitation. The agency had come a long way since nixing the CCC pentamidine proposal less than two years earlier because it was too novel.

While NIAID was reviewing the stack of applications, Mathilde Krim's American Foundation for AIDS Research was preparing to make its own contribution to community-based research. In April 1989, AmFAR gave fifteen organizations start-up grants totalling $1.4 million to begin local trials.

In July the County Community Consortium and the Community Research Initiative sponsored a joint conference on community-based research, held at Columbia University. Here, too, the mood was more conciliatory than combative; there was a race to the podium to praise the concept of grassroots research.

Representatives from blue-chip pharmaceutical companies talked about their commitment to fund local trials. Tony Fauci took the microphone to proclaim community research "totally compatible" with the mission of the National Institutes of Health and pledged to back it. Food and Drug Administration officials also jumped on the bandwagon of praise.

In October 1989, Health Secretary Louis Sullivan announced the NIAID community trial winners. By then Congress had upped the ante, making $9 million available to eighteen different programs. The accompanying press release seemed to have come straight from the mouths of AIDS activists. Tony Fauci said in the release: "We can take advantage of the extraordinary expertise of doctors in private practice, in community clinics and at large inner-city hospitals. These doctors are on the frontlines of the AIDS epidemic, and are involved in the day-to-day management of people infected with the AIDS virus."

Along with New York, San Francisco, and several other big cities with vocal gay populations, community trial sites were funded in Detroit, New Haven, New Orleans, and Newark, which all had severe drug-abuse problems and sizable minority populations infected with HIV. Selected sites included city hospitals, community clinics, private-physician consortia, health maintenance organizations, and drug treatment centers. The structure of each program reflected in part the population being served; the methadone maintenance clinic in East Harlem looked very different from the clinic designed to meet the needs of HIV-infected patients in the East Los Angeles barrio. Different still were the agencies serving the gay white male population in San Francisco's Castro District and a Navajo reservation in Arizona.

Along with having licensed doctors and nurses available to provide primary care, the NIAID grant required only that funded organizations be able to reach a great many HIV-infected persons and know how to care for them; to demonstrate strong community support; and to be well integrated into the local medical care system. Two-year contracts labeled Stage I were awarded to agencies without much background in community-based research; as part of their grant monies, the novices were to be trained in the art of writing protocols and the science of conducting clinical studies. More experienced agencies were given greater autonomy through Stage II contracts, which were each to last five years and gave them a fairly free hand in conducting research.

The awards announcements included one unexpected development: neither CRI nor some of the other early pioneers of the community-based movement were on the winner's list.

Not surprisingly, there was a lot of complaining about those omissions. Some people thought the decision was overtly political; CRI, in particular, had been highly critical of NIAID and its approach to research.

Others suggested CRI had grown careless. The whispered talk was that the pioneers of community-based research had become complacent, so convinced of the merits of their own work that they hadn't focused enough attention on producing a quality proposal. Indeed, subsequent events revealed deep flaws in the organization.

The day the grantees were announced, CRI was up in arms. Michael Callen fired off a note to NIAID demanding to know why his group had been excluded.

Three weeks later he got back a detailed debriefing letter signed by L. S. Pollack, chief of NIAID's contract management branch, and Lawrence Deyton, known to all as "Bopper," who headed the community research program. Although the letter was phrased politely, its contents were devastating.

NIAID officials told CRI its proposal failed to demonstrate that it could design and conduct clinical trials. They claimed CRI had spent too much time generalizing about the philosophy of community-based trials and not enough substantiating its own strengths. Previous research efforts were termed "inadequate," and CRI was criticized for failing to establish a solid outreach program within minority communities. In a final blow, NIAID questioned Bernie Bihari's leadership abilities and his experience in managing HIV-infected patients. Although the Harvard-trained Bihari's credentials in the field of alcoholism and drug dependency were impeccable, his administrative skills raised some concerns. In fairness, though, Bihari had conducted HIV-related clinical research since the mid-1980s as a member of the faculty at Downstate Medical Center in Brooklyn and as a physician with a part-time practice managing AIDS patients.

Despite the letter's conciliatory final statement—that CRI might have been awarded a grant had additional funds been available— Bihari and Ronald English, president of the board of directors, were furious.

In a fifteen-page response, they called the NIAID letter an outrageous document, a cover-up "full of lies, distortions, and half-truths," and "a sloppy and transparent" justification for a wrongheaded decision. They provided a point-by-point rebuttal to NIAID's charges.

Most damning was CRI's accusation that politics and personality had played a decisive role in the decision to deny the grant. Bihari and English said CRI was being punished for its noisy criticisms of the government's research system, and claimed NIAID wanted to bring the network of community-based research agencies entirely under its control. Another angry charge was that Margaret Fischl, who chaired the committee that had made the final selections, resented criticisms levied against her in the past by Joe Sonnabend. Sonnabend had been particularly enraged by—and publicly critical of—Fischl's placebo-controlled Bactrim trial, which had been published the year before. "It would be hard to imagine that she would not be influenced by Dr. Sonnabend's association with CRI," read the letter.

The insult to CRI, wrote Bihari and English, leaves us "no choice but to become the conscience of the AIDS research movement and to expose the shortcomings of the current system without pulling punches or being diplomatic. We regret this development, but, given the disastrous history of the AIDS Program, are not surprised that NIAID has made another major mistake."

Despite its determination to fight back, CRI never became a thorn in NIAID's side.

By 1990, many community physicians were alienated by the centralized research in CRI's 26th Street headquarters. Its top-heavy administrative structure was clearly impeding program development. Millions of dollars in research grants had been provided by the drug companies and by AmFAR, but no results had ever been published in a credible medical journal, not even the results of its historic pentamidine trials. Given its potential—it was in the city with the largest caseload in the country and had a vast number of doctors who saw patients in private practice—CRI was a major disappointment to its early supporters. Jay Lipner called it "a bad version of an ACTG," and ACT UP began a campaign to restructure the agency that was once such a rising star.

Bernie Bihari was ousted from his post as executive director at the end of the year, although he remained a lead investigator for the organization. Fiscal troubles continued, and in August 1991, CRI closed its doors. But the pioneer of community-based research intended to emerge with renewed vigor; as 1992 dawned, plans to launch the Community Research Initiative on AIDS, at the same location and involving many of the same people, were under way.

Despite CRI's troubles, community-based research continues to blossom.

With Don Abrams at the helm, CCC is flourishing, conducting its own trials and using NIAID's community research grant monies. A year after the awards were made, the eighteen NIAID sites launched their first trial, a study of two drugs to prevent toxoplasmic encephalitis, a life-threatening infection of the central nervous system. Although 50 percent of all adults are estimated to be infected by *Toxoplasma gondii*, a protozoan carried by cats that causes the disease, only people with severely depressed immune systems are likely to sicken or die.

AmFAR's commitment to grassroots trials also grew steadily. By the end of 1991, $5.6 million had been made available in seed grants to thirty-one centers around the country. More significantly, AmFAR and NIAID managed to overcome scientific rivalries, effectively joining forces to share data and to sponsor joint conferences.

Community-based trials have become as much a tool of empowerment as an approach to research. Patient and physician input is typically solicited during the design phase. While traditional trials frequently exclude patients taking other medications, community-based trials generally allow their use, so long as patients are frank about them. Confident that their admissions will not disqualify them, patients are less likely to lie—and consequently, study results are more likely to reflect real-life patient behavior outside the confines of clinical research.

Furthermore, because of their convenient locations, community-based organizations developed a much better track record than ACTG sites for enrolling women, minorities, and drug users. Access to ACTG trials remains limited to patients fortunate enough to live close to a testing site or willing to travel long distances at their own expense, which means losing their social and emotional support systems.

But locally based research is not about to replace big-ticket trials altogether. Some therapies do not readily lend themselves to testing in a community setting, especially the ones that involve costly technology, complicated medical procedures, or intense patient monitoring. Most ACTG sites are better equipped with sophisticated machinery and employ more researchers skilled in evaluating complex data.

Grassroots trials, important though they are, are likely to complement research in traditional settings, not replace it. One of the great unmet needs of the epidemic has been for small-scale, rapid tests on scores of promising therapies. Community-based research is ideally suited to that purpose. Also, by focusing on drugs to prevent or treat opportunistic infections or the debilitating wasting syndrome—which results from the body's inability to absorb food and leads to terrible diarrhea and dramatic weight loss—community research promises to extend life while the long vigil for a cure continues.

"We need to use the special expertise of both groups," said Mathilde Krim. "The ACTGs are best at doing high-tech research. But the community-based trial system is cheap, and when it comes to looking at patient tolerance and efficacy in the real world, they are the best. Community-based trials are here to stay."

If a cure for AIDS is ever found, if the scourge is someday relegated to the history books, community-based trials will likely remain as one of the epidemic's enduring legacies. Because it empowered patients and fostered strong ties with their physicians, community-based research offered, above all else, something whose value could not be measured: a sense of hope.

11

Business as Usual

The Patenting and Pricing of AZT

> EDWARD R. MURROW: Who owns the patent on this
> vaccine?
> JONAS SALK: Well, the people, I would say. There is no
> patent. Could you patent the sun?
>
> —"See It Now,"
> April 12, 1955

BURROUGHS WELLCOME was at the center of a furious storm over
pricing policies from the moment AZT was approved. Although its
price was slashed by 20 percent by the end of 1987, the drug still cost
patients an outrageous $8,000 a year.

In early 1989, sparks flew. Burroughs Wellcome had been stone-
walling congressional committees and mounting activist pleas to
lower its price and the demands were growing louder. Then, in August of that year, two of the largest AIDS trials ever conducted
showed that AZT could slow the progression of disease among some
infected people. Suddenly the size of the market for AZT exploded
exponentially. The stakes were higher than ever.

THE INVASION OF BURROUGHS WELLCOME

In January 1989, ACT UP's Peter Staley and Mark Harrington were on their way to Burroughs Wellcome's headquarters in North Carolina for a meeting with four top corporate officials.

Harrington and Staley are a curious and complementary duo. Where Staley is systematic and calm, Harrington is intense, smoking cigarette after cigarette and talking in rapid-fire sentences. Like so many other activists, Harrington became a public figure almost against his will, propelled into the forefront of political activism by the demands of the epidemic.

Until the mid-1980s, the wiry San Francisco native had knocked around quite a bit, mostly without a clear focus. After graduating from Harvard University with a degree in German art and film, Harrington lingered for a few years in Cambridge, where he worked as a waiter and occasional free-lance writer. Then he moved to New York City and soon signed on with ACT UP. AIDS brought him a purpose at last. Harrington was suddenly quoted regularly in the *New York Times* and other media and asked to speak before august national bodies.

Harrington and Staley had a message to deliver to BW that winter day, one the company was not going to enjoy hearing. The activists were ushered into the office of David Barry, Burroughs Wellcome's vice-president of research.

Harrington was the first to speak, and he was blunt: "People are being driven into poverty to pay for your drug. People who lack access are dying because they can't get your drug." Right to the point and never mind the small talk.

Barry struggled to keep the meeting cordial. He talked to the men about how important it was to earn sufficient revenues to sustain the company's research effort.

Staley and Harrington were not impressed by his remarks, which came as no surprise. Harrington's retort was sharp. "It's very ironic that the company which produces the first approved, effective treatment for this disease is held in universal hatred and disdain because of their pricing structure and their being very close-mouthed about what the justification for that cost is," he said.

Barry denied that the company's profits were excessive, and

claimed that the cost of AZT represented a relatively small proportion of the total price of care for an AIDS patient. He kept returning to the need for healthy profits. "I believe strongly that the answers to the major problems are going to come from the private, research-intensive pharmaceutical companies, and we have to be an example in every way. If we can't show that we're making money on it . . . there's either going to be fewer companies involved or less of an effort."

Soon other company representatives attending the meeting picked up the ball from Barry and began boasting about their patient-assistance program, which allowed eligible patients to receive AZT without charge. The activists exchanged skeptical looks; they knew about that program, which was run through the company's public-relations department and was notorious for its capricious eligibility criteria. Mark Harrington called it "a fig-leaf program." Staley criticized it as nothing more than a PR stunt.

The angry retorts ended the meeting on a bitter note. Burroughs Wellcome's only concession that day was to admit that the patient-assistance program's guidelines might be flawed and to agree to consider revisions.

Months passed. Despite repeated telephone calls to headquarters, the company made no move to restructure the program. And the price of AZT remained unchanged.

Although no tangible results emerged from the meeting, Peter Staley didn't leave Burroughs Wellcome entirely empty-handed. If nothing else had been accomplished, he'd at least been able to take a good look inside corporate headquarters. A daring idea was forming in his head, an idea bold enough to sound foolhardy, but if it worked, the pharmaceutical giant would surely take notice. Staley was hatching a plan to invade Burroughs Wellcome.

The drama began to unfold on Sunday, April 23, 1989, when nine ACT UP members piled into a rented van and drove from New York City to Durham, North Carolina. The invasion team called itself the Power Tools, its assignment, Mission Impossible. The crack commandos arrived at their destination late that evening and checked into the Durham Motel, squeezing themselves into three rooms.

Stuart Fisher, a local attorney whose involvement in political causes dated back to the 1960s, had earlier agreed to represent the nine men on a pro bono basis. At their motel, he laid out the possible

consequences of the planned action in no uncertain terms. If they
proceeded with their plans for an invasion, and if Burroughs Wellcome decided to play tough, every participant faced the risk of ten
years in prison. The invasion team listened attentively. They had
come too far to turn back now. Sure, there were risks, but they had
to be taken. Fisher's grim warning prompted no change in plans.

Tuesday morning, April 25, 1989. The men awoke early and
donned jackets and ties. They looked corporate and felt nervous.
Strategy was reviewed one final time. Four men were to penetrate
BW headquarters, three would remain outside to monitor the situation as it developed, and two would stay at the motel to handle the
expected barrage of press inquiries. The four men on the frontlines of
the invasion carried briefcases packed with cellular telephones,
walkie-talkies, handcuffs, chains, high-power drills, a variety of hardware, extra battery packs, and enough food and water to last three
days. A pocket-sized television set was also squeezed in—so the
Power Tools could watch themselves on the news.

From his previous North Carolina trip, Peter Staley knew the team
would have to get past a security desk in the building's front lobby.
The problem was, he hadn't quite figured out how to accomplish that.
The team decided to make a preliminary foray inside the target
building, hoping for inspiration. Staley pretended to have an appointment with a company employee and asked the uniformed guards
where the office was located. He was directed to another building,
but not before he managed to spot a bathroom at one end of the
lobby, past the security desk and close to the bank of elevators.

Now Staley knew how the Power Tools would strike.

A few minutes later the men returned to the security desk. After
telling guards they were unable to find the official with whom they
had an appointment, one of the Power Tools asked for permission to
use the bathroom.

The urge to go suddenly became contagious, and the guards waved
all four men through. Maybe it was fate; perhaps it was a simple
stroke of luck. But just as the Power Tools approached the elevator
banks, a door slid open. The team moved quickly inside, catching the
security force unprepared. One guard shouted out, "No. Wait." Time
stood still for one long moment as another passenger put her hand out
to open the door, thinking someone must be running for the elevator.

But seeing no one approach, she allowed the door to close again before the guard had moved from his desk. The assault had begun.

Next came occupation. Once upstairs, the men sought out an office facing the highway; earlier, they had decided that was preferable to an office overlooking the private parking lot, just in case Burroughs Wellcome decided to bar the press from its property. Inside one room, a woman sat alone at her desk talking on the telephone. With their walkie-talkies in hand, the men looked convincingly like security guards.

"Excuse me, ma'am. We have an emergency situation in this part of the building. Could you please go to the lobby?"

The ruse worked. The woman spoke hurriedly into the phone. "Marge, I've got to go, it's an emergency," she said, and dashed out of her office.

Within minutes, the Power Tools had used their drill and hardware to seal themselves inside. Only then did they encounter the first crimp in their plans. There were glass vents above the doors that had to be covered to make the office impenetrable. A solution was improvised by prying the backing off metal bookcases and securing it over the vent windows. Then they tried to unfurl their banner—which read, "Burroughs Wellcome's AZT: Pay or Die"—from the window to give the media a good photo opportunity. Instead, they encountered the only real disappointment of the day: the sealed windows proved indestructible and could not be smashed. Even hurling chairs against them proved fruitless.

Still, the moment was the culmination of weeks of planning. The team felt proud. It was time to share their victory with the men waiting on pins and needles outside the building. Staley picked up a walkie-talkie and said to the support team, "We're in, hit the media."

Some members of the national press had been alerted in advance, but to avoid a leak, local reporters were kept in the dark until the eleventh hour. Now word spread that men were holed up inside BW headquarters. Television crews and newspaper reporters converged on the scene, where they were able to interview the demonstrators via their cellular telephones. The ACT UP invaders were ready with two demands: a 25-percent drop in the price of AZT and a genuine corporate subsidy for those without resources or insurance to pay for the drug.

BW security was not sitting still through all this activity. Uniformed guards were on the scene within a few minutes. First the inside telephone lines were cut off. That only underscored ACT UP's foresight in bringing along a private communications system.

Then the Durham County sheriff arrived, and deputies began pounding with sledgehammers at the thin office walls where ACT UP was barricaded. Inside, the walls began to sway. Fine dust sprayed the room like a snowstorm. Moments before a human-size hole was punched through the wall, the Power Tools pulled out their chains and strapped themselves to the radiator. A red-faced sheriff finally pushed inside, breathing heavily, and pulled roughly at the men. Once it was clear there would be no violence, the sheriff calmed down. Within a few minutes the men were cut free from the radiator and led outside the building, still chained to one another, past the hordes of press people and off to the police station.

One of ACT UP's biggest concerns was that the media would portray it as a terrorist organization. But the fears proved ill-founded. After being released on $5,000 bail each, the Power Tools held a press conference on the courthouse steps and emphasized that property damage had not been their goal. As a show of good faith, they pledged to pay Burroughs Wellcome for any and all damages incurred. The day's event was at the top of the local news that night, and coverage was mostly sympathetic. Even the sheriff was quoted as saying that the men were some of the nicest people he'd ever arrested. Burroughs Wellcome eventually handed ACT UP a bill for $9,700 in damages. The amount was paid in full.

But the activists were less cooperative about returning to North Carolina to face criminal charges. Staley vowed that if the company chose to prosecute, the trial would become a major news event. Having had firsthand experience with ACT UP's media skills, Burroughs Wellcome knew the pledge was no bluff. The company asked the sheriff's department to drop all charges, and the Power Tools never set foot in a North Carolina courtroom.

EXPANDING THE AZT MARKET

For all the passion and drama it generated, AZT was initially recommended only for some 40,000 people—those with CDC-defined

AIDS. By the summer of 1989 the potential market for the drug mushroomed and the terms of the pricing debate began to shift.

First, Margaret Fischl announced the results of ACTG Protocol 016. The placebo-controlled study, in which neither researchers nor patients knew who was getting the active drug, was targeted at HIV-infected people who had early and mild symptoms of disease. And it clearly showed that AZT could slow progression to AIDS. Fischl's findings meant that at least 100,000 people, and perhaps twice that number, were likely to benefit from the drug.

Then preliminary findings from Protocol 019, the largest AIDS trial ever conducted, were released. Protocol 019 had been designed to determine the value of AZT in HIV-positive individuals with no symptoms at all. It was one of the most closely watched trials in history. Paul Volberding of San Francisco General Hospital was the principal investigator. The results were dramatic. When the trial demonstrated the drug could stop or slow progression to AIDS, at least half a million patients—those who were infected with the virus and had CD4 cell counts below 500—suddenly stood to benefit from AZT. With twice that number already infected, there would be plenty of others to follow.

Protocol 019 began just a few months after AZT was approved, and eventually enrolled 3,200 patients at thirty-two different medical centers around the country. One-third of the patients were given placebos, one-third got 500 milligrams of AZT, which was considered a low dose, and the last group got 1,500 milligrams, 300 milligrams more than the officially recommended dose for AIDS patients. Research subjects in each of the three arms were further divided into those with CD4 cells below 500 and those with higher counts.

Researchers monitoring the data said patients with the lower CD4 cell counts who were on placebo were twice as likely to develop AIDS as those getting either of the two doses of AZT. The blindfold was stripped from the study at once so that all subjects could get AZT.

The findings from 019 were considered enormously exciting. Suddenly there was firm evidence that HIV's march of destruction through the immune system could be halted or at least slowed. A press conference was immediately scheduled. "Today we are witnessing a turning point in the battle to change AIDS from a fatal disease to a treatable one," proclaimed Health Secretary Louis Sullivan before a swarm of reporters on August 17.

Just three days later, Barbara Arzymanow, a stock analyst with Kleinwort Benson Securities, predicted that per-share earnings of Burroughs Wellcome stock would skyrocket: "We are not talking significant increases here; we are talking quantum leaps."

She was right on the money. Within a month, the value of Burroughs Wellcome stock had soared 43 percent—and 32 percent of that increase came on August 18, one day after the press conference.

The result of Protocol 019 was not published for more than three years after the trial began. The lag raised important issues about how medical information is communicated to patients and their doctors.

The academic tradition for advancing basic science and the practice of medicine is to publish an article in one of a handful of prestigious journals. In a process that frequently takes years, data is first collected in lengthy studies, then it is analyzed and written up. Before a journal will accept it, the finished piece must be circulated for peer review. Historically, authors have been barred from talking about their findings until the publication date, although most journals have waived that rule for AIDS.

The theory behind the protracted process is sound; it is meant to ensure that only scientifically valid findings get aired in public. But publishing delays also result in treatment delays. And AIDS patients and their physicians haven't been willing to wait.

Years before Protocols 016 and 019 were completed, some doctors in private practice advised their patients without symptoms to take AZT, despite concerns about the drug's toxic side effects. In the absence of published research, this was highly controversial because no one really knew how and when to use the drug. Doctors played a guessing game in a practice that came to be known as "T-cell numerology." One physician prescribed low doses of AZT when a patient's CD4 cell count fell below 500. Another used 200 as the cutoff point. Still other physicians adopted altogether different criteria, either waiting until the CD4 cell count took a nosedive or simply leaving the decision in the patient's hands.

The results of Protocol 019 officially showed that the early use of AZT was a good idea. But more than 2½ years elapsed between the start of Protocol 019 and the press conference at the end of the trials. Another eight months dragged by until the studies were written up and the *New England Journal of Medicine* published the formal results in April 1990. During that time, doctors and patients who were not part of an insider's circle did not have any way to know that AZT was being used in asymptomatic patients. In rural America and among patients without access to state-of-the-art health care, AZT was prescribed only for the narrow population for whom the drug had originally been approved. Equally disturbing, few health insurance plans would pay for unproven uses of the exorbitantly expensive new drug until the FDA had officially approved AZT for use in asymptomatic, HIV-infected people.

Another inequity of the American health care system had been laid bare by the AIDS calamity.

After the August 1989 conference, the BW gold mine seemed bottomless. The market was not in the United States alone. If the drug was sold in the Third World—and if anyone could afford to buy it—tens of millions of people might want it. The staggering projections of sales further inflamed the volatile debate over the price. More people began to attack Burroughs Wellcome. In a speech to the American Association of Physicians for Human Rights, an association composed mostly of gay doctors, Tony Fauci said the drug manufacturer should be pressured to bring down the price of AZT. The *New York Times* jumped into the fray, calling the cost "astoundingly high" and "inhuman" in a lead editorial published on August 28. "Burroughs Wellcome is the subsidiary of a British company that is 75 percent owned by a charitable foundation, the Wellcome Trust. Wellcome's trustees are academics, many of them retired, who distribute the revenues for medical research. This is no doubt a worthy cause. But it's a strange kind of charity that cordons off people already suffering from a terrifying disease."

Congressman Henry Waxman came down hard on T. E. Haigler, then the company president. "The continued high price of the drug now appears to be an attempt to charge whatever patients, governments, and insurers can scrape together because they are desperate and have no alternative," wrote Waxman in a letter to Haigler. He added that the price seems "particularly inappropriate in light of the generous Federal assistance given to the company in the development, approval and marketing of the drug."

And then he issued a clear warning: "Burroughs Wellcome Company was given every benefit of every doubt that its price was necessary to continue research and development efforts and that only reasonable returns would be expected over the lifetime of the product. Few such doubts remain now, and we cannot continue to allow your pricing policies to go unexamined."

BW was also under pressure from a national alliance of AIDS organizations who had come together earlier that summer. In a statement on AZT pricing, the consortium called for "a dramatic reduction in price" as well as reauthorization of a federal program that subsidized AZT. Both steps were necessary, according to the statement, "if AZT is to do the good it can; if AZT is to be more than hope cruelly waved before hundreds of thousands of Americans with HIV infection."

Within a week of getting that message, Burroughs Wellcome called Jean McGuire, executive director of the AIDS Action Council, an umbrella organization of community-based groups from around the country formed to lobby on behalf of AIDS patients. The company suggested getting together for a meeting.

Jean McGuire was joined at the BW meeting by Peter Staley of ACT UP. Both assumed the company was ready to talk about lowering its price. Instead, officials merely repeated past promises to "review" costs at some vague future date.

By the time they met, the public flogging of BW had attracted a lot of interest from the press. Reporters waited eagerly outside the doors of the meeting to find out whether there had been some sort of a handshake deal. The company declined to elaborate on the outcome, with spokeswoman Kathy Bartlett saying only, "We consider this a private meeting where we hoped to have a frank exchange of information."

The patient advocates spoke more freely about their disappointments. McGuire told reporters that BW had offered nothing but "old rhetoric."

Staley complained of bad faith, noting, "They kept telling us why they needed all this money. But we left the meeting empty-handed."

He added, "We are on an adversarial path with this company."

ACT UP was used to playing an adversarial role, but this time the statement bore the weight of almost the entire activist community.

A multi-front attack was launched on Burroughs Wellcome. Lambda Legal Defense headed a legal committee to see whether grounds existed to challenge BW's exclusive patent. A legislative committee, led by representatives of the AIDS Action Council and the Gay Men's Health Crisis, was formed to explore the patent issue with Congressman Ted Weiss. Around-the-clock picketing was organized at the company's North Carolina headquarters, and stickers reading "AIDS Profiteer" were printed up and pasted on store displays of BW's over-the-counter pharmaceutical products. Momentum began to build for a nationwide boycott of BW products, which included Actifed and Sudafed, popular cold remedies.

ACT UP RETURNS TO WALL STREET

The heart of New York City's financial district was familiar territory to ACT UP. The group's first demonstration in March 1987 had spurred Staley into activism. A year later, protestors came back, with many more bodies but essentially the same complaints.

Now, in the fall of 1989, ACT UP was back for its third Wall Street engagement. This time, Peter Staley's experience as a bond trader came in handy.

The activists staked out the New York Stock Exchange like a crack commando unit. To reconnoiter the trading floor, they mingled in the visitor's gallery, where Yippie leader Abbie Hoffman had tossed down dollar bills twenty years earlier to dramatize his opposition to capitalism. Outside the Stock Exchange Building they posed as tourists while eyeing the security system, and noticed there was no metal detector.

One of the advance scouts carried a video camera with a macro-zoom lens and shot footage of the identification badges worn by the traders and clerks. The videotape was handed over to a graphic artist who duplicated the typeface and design of the badges. Assumed trader names and false identification numbers were used, with Bear Stearns listed as employer. The counterfeit badges were taken to a novelty shop in Greenwich Village, where they were encased in laminated plastic for eight dollars apiece.

Several days prior to the planned action, the interlopers clipped the false badges to their business suits and executed a trial run. Five minutes before the opening bell, they swept past the security guards in a sea of traders and were on the floor without anyone noticing. It was surprisingly easy. Pads and pencils in hand, they walked briskly about in search of an appropriate staging ground for the planned protest. The visitors' gallery would have been the easiest choice, but plate glass—installed after Hoffman's notorious prank—now separated it from the traders below. Operating from the floor itself was considered too risky. Finally, the ideal site was spotted—an open landing up a flight of steps near the building entrance, where VIPs were usually brought to survey the exchange floor.

Everything seemed to be in order, but as the ACT UP team was preparing to leave, there was suddenly a heart-stopping moment.

An older gentleman approached Staley, peered at his badge, and asked, "What kind of a number is that?"

"I don't know," Staley answered nervously. "I just got it."

The man hesitated for a fraction of a second, then thrust out his hand and said, "Welcome to the Exchange." Staley's sigh of relief was palpable as the man disappeared into the trading floor crowd.

He was perplexed by the question and wisely decided to investigate further. Soon he discovered that there were fewer than 1,400 members of the New York Stock Exchange—and his badge was numbered 4,263. That evening there was a frantic last-minute effort to redo the badges with numbers less likely to arouse suspicion.

The next day, Thursday, September 14, 1989, seven men met for breakfast at a McDonald's in the Financial District. After reviewing strategy one final time, they walked from the restaurant toward the New York Stock Exchange, stopping a block away to synchronize their watches. Staley took a few deep breaths. Then they divided into two groups, one entering the building at 9:25 A.M., the other precisely three minutes later.

Four guards were posted at the entrance but the ACT UP members passed by unchallenged. Two of those assigned to photograph the event split off while the other five infiltrators walked briskly up the staircase to the VIP landing. Within fifteen seconds, one ACT UP member had extracted a large chain from the money belt tucked in the back of his pants and looped it through the bannister. Then the demonstrators reached for the handcuffs in their pockets and locked themselves to the chain. A banner reading "Sell Wellcome," which had been stuffed down the front of one man's shirt, was unfurled. Seconds before the 9:30 A.M. opening bell, the activists began to blare portable foghorns, drowning out the signal. Fake $100 bills imprinted with the words "Fuck your profiteering. We die while you play business" were tossed to the traders below.

Staley recalled that moment with obvious satisfaction.

"Our intention was to be totally confrontational and antagonistic," he said. The crowd responded in kind, many tossing wads of paper at the demonstrators and yelling, "Kill the faggots," and "Mace the faggots." Within ninety seconds the first group of security guards arrived on the scene and confiscated the banners and foghorns. But the men, chained to the bannister, could not be budged. The guards had to scurry for a chain cutter. Staley had a moment to reflect on the situation and recalled his sense of triumph. "I knew we had succeeded totally. No matter how they screamed and shouted, it was we who would be at the top of the news that night."

A runner positioned outside the Exchange was handed two rolls of film from the photographers and raced the shots up to the Associated Press offices in midtown; the AP photo department had already been put on alert. The photographs were transmitted over the wires even before police arrived to lead the demonstrators out of the building.

THE BATTLE FOR THE AZT PATENT

The Wall Street demonstration, the scathing editorials in the *New York Times* and elsewhere, and Henry Waxman's threat to hold congressional hearings on the price of AZT put Burroughs Wellcome on the defensive. Four days after the invasion of the Stock Exchange, the company announced a 20-percent drop in the price of AZT, to $6,500 a year per patient, the second such cut it had been forced to make.

The move was not dictated by the laws of capitalism; in a free-market economy, BW was legally entitled to charge whatever it wished. Nor was it a matter of public image; the company's previous record clearly showed it wasn't terribly concerned about that. Rather, it was an indication that political pressures had become too intense for the company to resist. And there may have been another factor. Burroughs Wellcome was probably eager for the furor to die down because it believed its patent on AZT—a patent worth hundreds of millions of dollars—was vulnerable.

Throughout its time of troubles, the company insistently put forth its own interpretation of AZT's development, taking its case to the press, Congress, and the American public. Everywhere it repeated the same story: BW had taken the risks, made the scientific advances, and paid for the research that brought AZT to the marketplace. In a deliberate and systematic fashion, the company dismissed the contributions of Jerome Horwitz, Sam Broder, Hiroaki Mitsuya, and other government and academic scientists. When challenges to the validity of BW's patent on AZT arose—as the company probably suspected they would—a long paper trail had been established to document the claim that it was singlehandedly responsible for AZT. In a letter published in September 1989 by the *New York Times*, T. E. Haigler, BW's president, wrote: "Had we been reluctant to direct the full force of our research, clinical development and manufacturing expertise on this disease, there would have been no treatment for desperate patients in 1986. We sped ahead with the pivotal clinical trial, funded by us, that established the effectiveness of Retrovir."

That letter sent Sam Broder, head of the National Cancer Institute, ballistic. Until then, he had been reluctant to do battle with Burroughs Wellcome, despite the company's repeated attempts to rewrite history. "My job is to alleviate death and suffering, not to engage in unnecessary or unproductive arguments with my collaborators," said Broder.

Now, though, he unleashed his frustrations. The rebuttal he fired off in response, which was signed by others at NCI and at Duke, was published a few weeks later:

> The September 16 letter from T. E. Haigler, Jr., president of the Burroughs Wellcome Company, was astonishing in both substance and tone. Mr. Haigler asserts that azidothymidine, or AZT, was essentially discovered and developed entirely by Burroughs Wellcome with no substantive role from Government scientists and Government-

supported research. This will be a surprise to the many men and women who have devoted their lives to working for the viral cancer program and developmental therapeutics program of the National Institutes of Health over the last 25 years. . . .

In a number of specific ways, Government scientists made it possible to take a drug in the public domain with no medical use and make it a practical reality as a new therapy for AIDS. It is unlikely that any drug company could have found a better partner than the Government in developing a new product.

One of Broder's particular sources of irritation, he would later explain, was BW's failure to acknowledge the dedication of so many government workers. "A lot of men and women spent their entire career doing very difficult jobs under very difficult conditions," he said. "They have devoted their whole life to make things like AZT a reality, and then not to be acknowledged, that's not right." Broder and Mitsuya have privately admitted they were somewhat naïve in their dealings with Burroughs Wellcome and feel they had been treated unfairly.

What began as a skirmish between Sam Broder and Burroughs Wellcome eventually erupted into open warfare, and other parties were pulled into the conflict. Legal experts, public health officials, and politicians all began investigating the possibility that Burroughs Wellcome's patent on AZT should be revoked. (See Appendix C for a comprehensive discussion of the legal challenge to the AZT patent.)

Typically, it was a grassroots effort that pushed the patent issue to the fore. The federal government, of course, could have devoted far more resources than could community organizations to challenging Burroughs Wellcome. But there was no one willing to do it. In the Bush Administration there was neither the leadership nor the political will to rein in a corporate violator of the public trust. At Sam Broder's insistence, the National Institutes of Health did hire outside counsel to probe the AZT patent issue, and it was determined that grounds for a legal challenge indeed existed. But NIH did not pursue the logical next step—actually filing a lawsuit—because no one was willing to run with that political football without support from the White House.

By default, the task instead fell mostly into the hands of one man,

Mickey Davis, a Cleveland law professor with special expertise in patent law. For the next year Davis sat in his Cleveland office, running up huge telephone and fax bills as he struggled to involve other interested parties and to establish the litigation team to contest the BW patent.

Meanwhile, other events were spinning out of BW's control. In Canada, two small generic drug manufacturers went on the offensive. First they filed their own challenge to the AZT patent, claiming the drug "was not an invention but merely the result of expected skill and a workshop improvement." That technical language essentially means that BW is making claims for the drug that are too wide, given the limitations of its patent. Then Apotex, one of the Canadian companies, began selling AZT to Interpharm Laboratories, an independent company based in the Bahamas, which put the drug in its mail-order catalogue, making it available to Americans and anyone else who wanted to order it. Interpharm priced its AZT at eighty-nine cents a capsule, about 35 percent less than the equivalent quantity in the United States.

By March 1991, thanks largely to Mickey Davis's persistence, the legal framework for the patent challenge in the United States was in place. The Washington-based Public Citizen Litigation Group filed a suit on behalf of the PWA Health Group, the New York buyers' club, and two HIV-infected people, claiming that BW's patent on AZT was invalid. Mickey Davis was named "of counsel" in that suit. Not surprisingly, the company's attorneys moved at once to dismiss that action, claiming a consumer-rights agency had no legal standing to question the validity of a patent. That suit is pending.

Two months after the Public Citizen suit was filed, Barr Laboratories, a small drug manufacturer in Pomona, New York, asked the FDA to approve its generic version of AZT, claiming it would sell the drug for half of BW's price. BW again took swift legal action, charging Barr with patent infringement in U.S. District Court. Barr promptly countersued and said that the National Institutes of Health should be named as coinventor of the patent. Although NIH did not directly participate in that suit, it agreed to license the drug to Barr if the company triumphed over Burroughs Wellcome and the government secured the patent for AZT. NIH also agreed to pay some of Barr's expenses and supply information to document its case. Bernadine

Healy, director of the National Institutes of Health, issued a press release that explicitly backed Barr's contention that NIH was entitled to share the AZT patent: "The intellectual and scientific contributions made by NCI to the evaluation of AZT were essential components of the invention of AZT therapy. . . . NIH believes that investigators at the National Cancer Institute should have been named coinventors on the AZT-related patents issued to Burroughs Wellcome." The BW/Barr suits are working their way through court.

With worldwide sales of AZT topping $1 billion by August 1991, the pressures on the company are intense. Taken together, the pending lawsuits and countersuits have raised a tangle of legal issues that will require a battalion of lawyers months—or, more probably, years—of toil to sort out. The company's claim in its patent application to have been the sole inventor of AZT rests at the heart of the dispute. In the eyes of Burroughs Wellcome, Jerome Horwitz's design skills, Sam Broder's prescience, Hiroaki Mitsuya's risk-taking, and all the laboratory work conducted at the National Cancer Institute and at Duke University apparently counted for naught.

12

ON THE DEFENSIVE

Pentamidine Profits and a Corporation Under Siege

To sell dearer or to buy cheaper than a thing is worth
is in itself unjust and unlawful.

—St. Thomas Aquinas

FOR ITS RESPONSIVENESS to government pleas to manufacture pentamidine and its willingness to underwrite the community-based trials that led to the approval of the drug, Lyphomed thought it would be portrayed as a white knight, giving hope and extended life to thousands of people with AIDS. The corporation also anticipated basking in the glow of praise from Wall Street's soothsayers. In May 1988, Lyphomed was already "on everybody's can't miss, high-growth stock list over the past five years," according to *Crain's Chicago Business*.

Instead the company became the target of FDA regulatory action and activist rage. Lyphomed became embroiled in the generic-drugs scandal that ripped at the fabric of the FDA, and the company was portrayed as a heartless profiteer by the press, some activists, and many political leaders. The company was also forced to the mat with

Fisons to protect its exclusive marketing rights to aerosolized pentamidine.

Just a year after the glowing *Crain's* prediction, the tables had turned sharply. A business reporter at the *Chicago Tribune* showed how far Lyphomed had fallen when he wrote that the once high flyer was now faced with "lost customers, lost sales, lost image and lost shareholder value." At the end of the decade, the makers of pentamidine found themselves battered on all fronts.

Lyphomed's woes began in the winter of 1987 when the FDA sent out a regulatory letter noting "significant violations" of good manufacturing practices at its plant in Melrose Park, Illinois. Forty-four different infractions were cited. The firm was also charged with illegally distributing pentamidine across state lines before filing the necessary paperwork with the FDA.

Lyphomed was told that no pending drug applications would be approved until it had restored a measure of quality control. A second FDA inspection at the Melrose Park plant a few months later showed things hadn't improved much. Lyphomed eventually closed down the Illinois facility rather than invest in necessary production improvements.

Soon after the Illinois violations came to light, the company faced almost identical charges in Orlando, Florida, where FDA inspectors seized its entire stock of injectable vitamins, nutrients, and other drugs. That plant was eventually shut down as well. In the interim, small-scale seizures took place at Lyphomed distribution sites in New Jersey, California, Georgia, and Texas.

At a stockholders' meeting in 1988 there were bitter complaints about Lyphomed's failure to disclose its skirmishes with the FDA. Dissatisfied by management's lack of response, a series of lawsuits were eventually filed against company officers. Ultimately, the firm paid $10 million to settle the claims outside of court.

But the troubles did not end there. While Lyphomed was fending off the FDA and its own stockholders, it was also coming under increasing attack for the price of pentamidine. In October 1984, when the FDA bestowed orphan drug status on Lyphomed's injectable pentamidine, the wholesale price stood at $25 for a 300-milligram

vial, enough for one month's supply. By the following year, when the
aerosolized version of the drug was shown to prevent the development of PCP in rats, the price was raised to $39.49. Then Lyphomed
filed an application to begin its first human trials on aerosolized
pentamidine and pushed the price to $54.79 in July 1986. In April
1987, as the trials continued, wholesale pentamidine was hiked another 28 percent, to $69.95. In August of that year, pentamidine shot
up again, this time to $99.45, where it remained until June 1991.

In all, the price increased 400 percent over a three-year period. An
AIDS drug once again became enmeshed in controversy over cost.
The company was accused of "needless and shameless price-goug-
ing" by more than one prominent researcher. At the turbulent stockholders' meeting, three AIDS activists were forcibly ejected from the
room after their complaints about pentamidine's high price grew
boisterous.

But they were not alone in deriding Lyphomed's policies. Congressional investigators claimed the company had seized on pentamidine
as a way to leap from the minor-league playing field of a small
generic-drug manufacturer straight to the majors. Ted Weiss demanded a justification for the price hikes and lashed out at Brian
Tambi, the corporation's president, when he testified before his congressional subcommittee in April 1988.

Weiss was blunt: "You saw a good thing which could be used to
build your company to a size you'd never anticipated. And how do
you pay for it? You pay for it by soaking the clientele. I think it is really
unfortunate."

Suddenly, just about everyone wanted a look at the company's
books.

After a few years of fiscal health in the mid-1980s, Lyphomed was on
shaky financial ground again. It lost $21 million in 1988; without
pentamidine, the figure would have been far higher. Its stock price
plummeted from a high of about $30 in 1987 to a fifty-two-week low
of less than $9 per share. One year later, while the company was still
fighting charges of profiteering, pentamidine was essentially floating
the company, accounting for almost 40 percent of the firm's total sales
of $165 million. The other 60 percent came from numerous other
products, including antibiotics, vitamins and other nutrients, cardio-

vascular drugs, steroids, and oncology drugs. Sales from one other AIDS drug—amphotericin B, used to treat cryptococcal meningitis— were also included in that 60 percent. Its side effects were often brutal, but when Lyphomed released some contaminated vials of the drug, the problem got a lot worse. The FDA began an investigation after patients using it experienced intense chills, and in January 1988, Lyphomed voluntarily recalled 20,000 vials of the drug.

Despite its tumbling public image and hefty losses, Lyphomed's board of directors managed to do quite well for themselves. Board Chairman John Kapoor had a contract, executed when he first joined the company in 1978, that gave him the right to buy Lyphomed. He exercised that option in 1981, using $2.7 million furnished almost entirely by venture capitalists and bonds, a mere $10,000 reportedly coming out of his own pocket. Later, Lyphomed went public and Fujisawa, one of Japan's largest pharmaceutical corporations, began eyeing the firm voraciously. The Osaka-based company already had some $1.6 billion in annual sales and was trying to make inroads into the American market.

Fujisawa's ambitions meshed perfectly with Lyphomed's needs. Having made its first profitable foray into the brand-name drug business with pentamidine, the company was looking for a substantial infusion of capital in order to transcend its identity as a small generic-drug manufacturer. The match was a natural.

In October 1986, Fujisawa purchased 30 percent of Lyphomed's stock. A standstill agreement barred the Japanese company from buying any more without board approval. Permission proved easy to get—once the board was assured its cut. John Kapoor orchestrated the deal, which proved so lucrative that he was accused of a "breach of fiduciary duties" by shareholders who filed a class-action suit against Kapoor, Lyphomed, Fujisawa, and other players in the take-over. In a related claim, company officials were accused of "aiding and abetting a conspiracy." Ultimately, the parties agreed in principle on a settlement that awarded the plaintiffs a maximum of $200,000 in attorneys' fees and another $40,000 in expenses. It was nothing that would derail the whole deal.

By September 1989, less than three months after Lyphomed received FDA approval to market aerosolized pentamidine, Fujisawa completed its takeover, paying an additional $640 million to acquire the remainder of the company, lock, stock, and barrel. Not bad for a small-town Illinois firm worth just over $2 million only eight years earlier.

Although Kapoor had gradually sold off much of the stock he'd owned when he took over the company, he still held a hefty 14 percent when the Fujisawa deal was consummated. He peddled his remaining 4.1 million shares to the Japanese and walked away with nearly $133 million in his pocket.

For the pharmacist from Bombay, it was an American dream ride to fame and fortune, and pentamidine was the ticket for the trip.

Despite price hikes and cashing in on the takeover deal, Lyphomed found common cause with some in the patient community. The National Organization for Rare Disorders paid tribute to Lyphomed at an annual awards banquet, where Commissioner Frank Young was also honored for his support of the Orphan Drug Act. Michael Callen commented: "I cannot say whether their price has been justified, but I can say that they were the first company to put its money down in a gamble on an experimental approach to AIDS treatment research and I believe that we have all won that gamble."

Still, Lyphomed had to spend a lot of time defending itself. Along with testifying before Weiss's committee, Lyphomed hired Geto & deMilly, a well-known Manhattan public-relations firm, to arrange a series of dog-and-pony shows with key academics, policymakers, and AIDS activists.

These round-table discussions were long and costly. Brian Tambi, Cynthia Yost, Lyphomed's director of marketing, and Bruce Montgomery, a physician who was involved in the early testing of pentamidine at San Francisco General, were there. So was Stuart Fisher, representing Geto & deMilly. The company's ace in the hole was the politically well-connected James Foster, one of the founding fathers of San Francisco's gay movement and a close adviser to Mayors George Moscone, Dianne Feinstein, and Art Agnos. Until his death from AIDS on Halloween, 1990, Foster served simultaneously as a health commissioner in San Francisco and a paid consultant to Lyphomed, hired to counter the harsh criticism being levied against the firm.

At Lyphomed's public-image booster meetings, Tambi cast the firm as a David surrounded by Goliaths. He took the battering personally, complaining, "It saddens us very much, after we have put so much of our lives into this work, morning, noon, and night, seven days a week, that there is so much misinformation, so much conjecture, so much anger which is turning into an ugly verbal assault on innocent people like myself."

Tambi added, "From the day it went to the rescue of the AIDS patient, this company has been in trouble."

To everyone who would listen, Tambi claimed the company had made no profit on pentamidine. Perhaps it would never do so, he alleged. The assertion, while not fully credible, was tough to challenge since the company refused to release its revenue and expense sheets on the drug. In fairness, that's standard operating procedure—Burroughs Wellcome also refused to make public its profits on AZT—but the absence of candor limited informed debate.

Lyphomed's top brass also claimed the price hikes on pentamidine largely reflected the fact that the initial price had been too low to cover unforeseen expenses. Tambi explained that generic-drug manufacturers lacked the administrative and R-and-D infrastructure, as well as the "deep pockets," of companies more experienced with brand-name products. He claimed Lyphomed had had to create, from scratch, an entirely new structure to market, sell, and support injectable pentamidine. Twenty physician salesmen, each paid more than $100,000 in salary and benefits, had been brought on board to educate the medical community on use of the new therapy. The FDA's decision to force aerosolized pentamidine through the maze of the full testing and approval process meant the company ran up bills totaling another $23 million. And post-approval studies required by the FDA were expected to cost the company $15 million more.

Jim Foster chimed in at the round-table discussion to sing the capitalist's refrain: "If a company doesn't make a profit consistently, it will not be around to make drugs for AIDS or anything else."

Tambi next touted Lyphomed's early willingness to produce injectable pentamidine when no other company would do so. "If the drug had enormous commercial potential, there would have been no need for the CDC and the FDA to seek out any company to make it, let alone a small generic company," Tambi pointed out.

He also reminded listeners that aerosolized pentamidine was not the only therapy, or even the most common one, used to treat or prevent PCP. Several other approved antibiotics remained the first lines of defense, and each one shrank the size of Lyphomed's potential market. Furthermore, Tambi said the exclusive rights to sell aerosolized pentamidine were largely illusory. He reasoned that since the seven-year Orphan Drug Act marketing exclusive on injectable pentamidine expired in 1991, other manufacturers would be permitted to sell the drug generically. Once that happened, Tambi was convinced that patients and physicians would purchase the product from other sources and aerosolize it themselves. For all practical purposes, nearly five years of orphan-drug exclusivity would thus be lost.

All in all, the top managers at Lyphomed appeared a disillusioned lot. In their view, they had played by the rules of the private enterprise game and were now being penalized for it. And as if they didn't have enough headaches, Lyphomed soon had to contend with the AIDS underground.

In September 1989 the PWA Health Group, the New York City buyers' club, held a press conference to announce its intention to import pentamidine from England, where it was available at a fraction of its American cost. Derek Hodel, the group's executive director, claimed it was an evolution of the FDA's "personal use policy," which had been developed the previous year to allow individuals to import limited quantities of drugs for noncommercial purposes. It marked the first organized effort by a buyers' club to import already approved medications solely because they were cheaper than the above-ground version.

The group's motivation was simple. "Because of the high U.S. price, many of those in need of this treatment simply do without," said Hodel. "Although pentamidine is available in this country, *it is not available enough.*"

To illustrate that point, Hodel talked about Carmen, a fifty-year-old single mother infected with HIV and at risk for PCP. Her job provided no health insurance but enough income to disqualify her from Medicaid. The medical clinic where she went for care was not equipped to administer pentamidine. The best advice her social worker could offer was to quit work to qualify for Medicaid. All her doctor could recommend was that she purchase a $200 nebulizer that allowed her to inhale the drug at home. Carmen could not afford either option. Instead, her pentamidine prescription went unfilled.

The idea for importing pentamidine was hatched at the annual international AIDS conference, held that year in Montreal, a few months before the press conference. That event is as much a pharmaceutical trade show as a scientific forum, with row after row of slick, industry-sponsored exhibits crammed with glossy brochures about new products, and with manicured salespeople eager to tout their wares. At the conference, Hodel visited the booth set up by Rhone-Poulenc, whose British subsidiary had originally supplied the Centers for Disease Control with pentamidine. Hodel asked casually about pricing policies and learned that pentamidine retailed in Canada for about $60 a vial. That was a startling revelation to Hodel, since it sold for almost $100 a vial in the United States at the time. "It had really never occurred to me that prices would be so different," said Hodel. "I hadn't any idea at that time how much they varied from country to country."

Hodel tried to purchase pentamidine from the Canadians, but negotiations with the manufacturer did not pan out. Then he made inquiries of pharmaceutical connections in England and discovered the price there was even lower—just $26 a vial, barely one-quarter of its cost in the U.S.

Hodel's move to import pentamidine and sell it cheaply was a direct threat to Lyphomed. The company responded as though a friend had stabbed it in the back, and moaned about betrayal. One executive asked, "How could they do this to us after all we've done for them?"

Tambi called the action shortsighted and said that patients had a personal stake in encouraging pharmaceutical companies to invest in AIDS therapies. "Limiting the return on such investments is not good public policy or in the best interests of the national AIDS community," he said.

Hodel sympathized with Lyphomed—up to a point. He admitted his actions put the company in a "terrible position" but boldly proclaimed that marketing rights could not take priority over patients' rights to life-saving medication. "Our position is that we don't really care what Lyphomed's problems are," said Hodel.

Lyphomed called the move a violation of the Orphan Drug Act and other federal codes, and fought back. Suddenly—and a bit incongruously, in light of its past manufacturing practice violations—quality control became the company's foremost concern. In an angry letter to the FDA, Tambi wrote: "The U.S. government cannot guarantee the safety and effectiveness of a drug produced in a foreign country if the drug has not met U.S. approval standards."

Brian Tambi also claimed that the FDA's personal-use policy applied only to drugs that had not yet been approved in the United States, and fired off a letter to Commissioner Frank Young, calling on him to stop the illegal importation of aerosolized pentamidine and "discourage those who circumvent the law."

Hodel disagreed with Tambi's interpretation and said the FDA's policy did not distinguish between approved and unapproved drugs.

At first the FDA was prepared to side with Tambi. Word was passed to Hodel that authorities were about to issue an import alert requiring U.S. Customs officials to seize pentamidine at the border.

Hodel called Jay Lipner and told him the import alert was coming. Lipner picked up the telephone and called Young. The document authorizing the alert was lying on the commissioner's desk awaiting his signature.

"Don't do this," Lipner told Young. "You're going to cause unbelievable grief to yourself and to everyone else if you do. Hold off until we can have a meeting."

Young agreed, and the date was quickly set. Two days later, Hodel flew down to Washington, along with Bill Rubenstein from the ACLU and David Barr from Lambda, to caucus with Young.

"Something was worked out," said Lipner with classic understatement. Whatever actually transpired behind closed doors, one thing is certain: no move was ever made to shut down the pentamidine operation. It continues to this day, allowing hundreds of people to purchase aerosolized pentamidine at local buyers' clubs as long as they have a physician's prescription. Buyers typically lack health insurance that covers prescription drugs adequately, or they have insurance but don't want their carrier, or an employer, to know they need the drug. Whichever is the case, they can't pay Lyphomed's charges out of their own pockets.

Until June 1991, Lyphomed's wholesale price had stood at just under $100 a vial, unchanged since its last price hike almost four years earlier. Since most pharmacists in high-incidence cities put only a small markup on the drug, people with AIDS were usually able to obtain it for between $105 and $175. In the hinterlands, though, where there was less competition, the price sometimes soared to $300 a vial.

Ultimately, Lyphomed made concessions to patient pressures and showed that its greed had limits. In June 1991, the company lowered the price of aerosolized pentamidine to $79, possibly hoping to generate some goodwill on Capitol Hill, where its windfall profits were still causing consternation. But even with the 20-percent cut, Lyphomed's drug was still overpriced. After customs and handling charges, underground pentamidine generally cost $40 a vial.

TURF WARS AND GOOD INTENTIONS

While the buyers' club was carving out one small piece of Lyphomed's pentamidine market, Fisons had not given up its attempts to secure a bigger chunk. The determined competitor had headed north to Canada to run its own trials while Lyphomed was underwriting community-based studies in New York and San Francisco. It made no secret of the reason why: in Canada, the drug was not easily available through private physicians, so patients were more willing to participate in a placebo-controlled trial where they had a 50-percent chance of getting the active drug. Fisons was harshly criticized for its naked expediency—but defended its decision as a reasonable response to FDA's demands for "pure" data.

Even when Lyphomed won the exclusive license for aerosolized pentamidine, Fisons refused to fade away. Several months after Lyphomed's drug was approved, Fisons handed its data to the FDA to be evaluated. Then the pharmaceutical giant began angling for the right to market its own product.

In theory, just one pharmaceutical company is allowed to sell an orphan drug for seven years after it is approved. Fisons, however, claimed that with help from Sloan-Kettering, it had developed a better nebulizer—a "clearly superior technology," said some researchers. They emphasized that a special advantage of the Fisons product was that it allowed lower doses of the drug to be used and was easier to use at home. Surely, said the company, the Orphan Drug Act was not intended to deny patients access to the best available product.

Eventually, Fisons took its case to Congress. Edward M. Bernard, a research associate at Sloan-Kettering, said: "If Congress fails to take action and the Lyphomed product retains exclusivity until 1996, we may be sentencing AIDS patients to less than the best available therapy for all those six long remaining years."

Not surprisingly, Brian Tambi violently opposed efforts to get the Fisons/Sloan-Kettering system on the market. In every public and private forum available to him, Tambi complained about how the rules were being changed midstream. "Tell us what the rules are and we'll play by them. But don't change the rules in the middle of the game. No rational person would make such an investment if there was no certainty as to the return that could be expected if the venture succeeded."

The whole point of the Orphan Drug Act had been to draw more companies into drug research unlikely to prove profitable. The fight between Lyphomed and Fisons highlighted one of the wrinkles in the act: Could a drug remain an orphan if it became attractive enough to have two parents fighting for its custody?

In the nine years since the Orphan Drug Act was passed, at least four orphan products had generated more than $100 million in annual sales and reaped unexpected bonanzas for their sponsors. AZT surpassed that high-water mark in 1988, and analysts believe that pentamidine went over the threshold in 1991.

The third drug in the same sales category is erythropoietin, known as EPO. It is approved to treat anemia associated with chronic kidney failure and sold as an orphan drug by Amgen, the California-based biotechnology firm. First-year sales were just over $302 million. EPO is also under study for AIDS-related anemia by Ortho Pharmaceuticals, a subsidiary of Johnson & Johnson, under a Treatment IND approved in June 1989. In 1989, conflicts over licensing rights left some AIDS patients enrolled in EPO trials without access to the drug for several months. The drug was eventually made available again and Amgen won its legal battle in 1991, but corporate profits continue to grow.

The fourth orphan drug is human growth hormone (HGH), used to

treat dwarfism in children. Genentech, located in South San Francisco, and Eli Lilly, based in Indianapolis, share the lucrative market
for two different versions of HGH. Estimated annual sales for Genentech are $200 million; Eli Lilly grosses $50 million.

Clearly, the original intent of the legislation had not been to line
the pockets of the pharmaceutical industry. But the Orphan Drug Act
had changed quite a bit since the first proposals were put forward in
1979. For example, one clause had originally required companies to
reimburse the government for any subsidies they received once drug
revenues reached some defined level. But in the final law, enacted in
the hands-off-industry climate that has prevailed during the Reagan
and Bush eras, the payback concept vanished. That dilution set the
stage for the abuses that would occur with so many AIDS drugs.

Another big change was orchestrated by industry lobbyists via
amendments after the act was passed. Initially, drug companies had
to disclose their R-and-D costs and document projected sales before
getting an orphan designation. Rather than laying bare their pricing
practices—which meant exposing the profitability of some rare-disease drugs to public scrutiny—the pharmaceutical industry fought for
revisions.

Eventually they got those revisions and the law was amended to
allow a drug to be designated an orphan if it was used to treat a
disease affecting fewer than 200,000 persons in the United States.
The number was somewhat arbitrary; the main point was that using
population targets rather than profit-and-loss figures meant the drug
companies did not have to worry about a government watchdog eyeing their ledger sheets. As a result, the concept of public accountabil-
ity in exchange for public subsidies got lost in the name of trade
secrets and free enterprise.

Coupled with widespread distress over pentamidine pricing and
the blockbuster sales of AZT, the spat between Lyphomed and Fisons
helped spotlight abuses of the Orphan Drug Act. Amid a building
chorus of criticism, Congressman Henry Waxman, the chief sponsor
of the 1983 legislation, held hearings to consider possible reforms. In
the spring of 1990, Waxman drafted amendments designed to curb
the unseemly profits possible under the Orphan Drug Act and ensure
that scientific innovation could still take place.

Under the Waxman proposals, the 200,000-person threshold was revised. To win orphan status on a drug, and thus lucrative incentives under the act, drug companies would have to project potential market size over a three-year period. The reform legislation would have revoked a company's exclusive rights to sell a drug the moment more than 200,000 people needed it.

Another amendment permitted two companies that had developed a drug at about the same time to share the seven-year marketing exclusive. The Lyphomed/Fisons dispute was foremost in the mind of legislators when that clause took shape. The Waxman amendments were designed to cut the profiteering out of the Orphan Drug Act.

Lyphomed stood to be the big loser if the 1990 Orphan Drug Act amendments passed. The other players who controlled $100-million orphans had already lobbied successfully for exemptions to the reform legislation. Genentech, one of the corporate powers behind human growth hormone, reportedly paid a team of lobbyists to help protect its market share. At least one hired gun was matched to every senator and congressman involved with the Orphan Drug Act amendments. Amgen also handed out big money to influential lobbyists to win protection from Congress.

But Lyphomed faced double trouble. First, 200,000 people already needed pentamidine or would soon, which meant its orphan-drug designation could be lost. Second, the provision for shared marketing rights would have allowed Fisons to break the lock on its monopoly. Lyphomed refused to give up its multimillion-dollar AIDS drug without a fight. Company lawyers circulated briefs to the Justice Department, key members of Congress, and the Department of Health and Human Services alleging that the Orphan Drug Act amendments represented a breach of contract and were unconstitutional.

As the fall congressional session was drawing to a close, in the early-morning hours of a Sunday in October, the 1990 Orphan Drug Amendments were passed unanimously by both houses. Lyphomed's strenuous lobbying helped get a "grandfather" clause that protected its exclusive marketing rights but the company remained disgruntled by the 200,000-person cap. In typical Washington style, Lyphomed tapped the old boys' network, hiring as its lobbyist the law firm of Bayless, Boland, Bates, and Madigan, which is littered with former assistants to George Bush and John Sununu, Bush's former chief of staff.

Along with the pressure Lyphomed was able to generate on the White House, President Bush and Vice-President Dan Quayle had their own reasons for disliking the amendments. Both men had close ties to Eli Lilly, whose stake in human growth hormone gave it an incentive to keep the Orphan Drug Act unchanged. Bush had once served on Lilly's board of directors and Quayle, who is from an old Indianapolis family, had received substantial campaign contributions from the company.

It was surely no coincidence that Bush exercised the right of a pocket veto a few weeks later, killing any chance of reform until the next congressional session. The Council on Competitiveness, an influential and highly conservative policy group chaired by Quayle, which is notorious for operating in secrecy and without consumer input, immediately issued a fact sheet to justify the veto. New legislation had to be introduced all over again.

In the meantime, the FDA took its own stand against abuses. The agency, which had been charged with administering the Orphan Drug Act when it first became law in 1983, had taken an astounding eight years to propose formal regulations. In January 1991, it finally put forth a proposal that would allow other companies to sell a drug chemically similar to an orphan product already on the market only if it could be shown to be safer or more effective than the existing product. The goal was to ensure that exclusive rights to market an orphan drug did not discourage the development of improved therapies. Unfortunately, however, the FDA's regulations did not limit the orphan-drug incentives only to products of "little commercial value"—there were still few holds barred on any company's right to reap extraordinary profits.

While the FDA was collecting comments on its proposal, Congress went back into session. On April 10, 1991, U.S. Representative Pete Stark of California took the podium to announce his proposed Orphan Drug Windfall Profits Tax Act. In introducing the legislation, Stark said, "Surely no one can argue that drug manufacturers should profiteer on the backs of the unfortunate few with rare diseases or medical conditions. But a handful of orphan drug makers somehow interpret or plan drug status as a license to profiteer."

Seven months later, just before the Thanksgiving recess, Kansas Senator Nancy Landon Kassebaum, who said the Orphan Drug Act had become "big business," and Ohio Senator Howard Metzenbaum seconded Stark's sentiment by proposing their own reform legislation. Their bill, which would rescind a company's market exclusivity on an orphan product once cumulative sales topped $200 million, was a dramatic attempt to curb the abuses of the act. The debate was beginning anew.

Brian Tambi believed the federal government had left a long trail of broken promises almost from the start in its dealings with the company. By late 1990, Lyphomed grew tired of sitting on the sidelines while its market was attacked from all directions. And so, in the tradition of merchants and marketing mavens everywhere, Lyphomed ran a "two-fer" sale.

It was done under the guise of a postmarketing study, but that was a chimera from the start. The real goal was to capture lost market share. An interoffice memorandum from Lyphomed to its hospital sales managers was explicit about that. The program, read the memo, "has been developed to recapture business lost to illicit pentamidine. . . . The program is intended to be used exclusively for accounts that we have lost to imported pentamidine."

Doctors who agreed to participate were given two vials of pentamidine for the price normally charged for just one, and Lyphomed's sales reps deliberately targeted physicians whose patients were getting the drug from buyers' clubs. "There really is no study. You don't have to give us data and we won't bother you about it," a Lyphomed representative told a physician point-blank.

The whole thing backfired on Lyphomed when the sham study was made public. Eight weeks after it was launched—without the most basic accouterments of a legitimate study, such as FDA approval, signed patient consent forms, or ethical review—Lyphomed called a halt to the whole thing and was publicly embarrassed.

13

ABSENCE OF VISION

The Ganciclovir Scandal

❖

I want to know where the leadership is from the
President. He lives in a different world than I do,
because he is not affected by AIDS. You know, I see
points of light also, but I see points of light because I
have CMV retinitis, not because I see a different
vision of America.

—JAY LIPNER,
lawyer and AIDS activist,
1945–1991

EVEN IF BURROUGHS WELLCOME had been an upstanding model of a
socially concerned corporation—which it most certainly was not—
AZT was no miracle cure. And for the thousands of patients who
could not tolerate it, time was running out. The cascade of AIDS
drugs that had been predicted to follow on its heels never material-
ized. Not until 1991, when ddI was approved, was a second antiviral
drug even on the market. Until then, people with AIDS had only
three choices when AZT's side effects became intolerable or the
immune system continued to decline. They could stop taking the drug
and await the consequences passively, they could plead to enter a
research study, or they could secure treatments from the AIDS underground.

The thirst for effective drugs remained unquenched. Activists and public health experts continued to look for new ways to reach two old goals: expanding access to unapproved drugs and identifying creative ways to get drugs to market even when the available data was incomplete or collected without traditional scientific rigor.

Nothing so dramatically illustrated the latter need as a virulent infection known as cytomegalovirus retinitis, the terror of blindness, and a man named Terry Sutton.

Cytomegalovirus retinitis, caused by an out-of-control herpes virus, is one of the cruelest diseases associated with AIDS. Some 20 percent of all people with AIDS face the horror of CMV retinitis. At first it may cause no symptoms, but the inflammation of the retina inevitably worsens until the brain can no longer interpret the signals it receives. Left unchecked, the disease invariably leads to blindness.

Syntex, a Palo Alto–based drug company, was the first to identify a drug that might suppress active CMV infection. Syntex synthesized ganciclovir in 1980, and it quickly established activity against a host of herpes viruses. Like AZT, ganciclovir was a nucleoside analogue, but its antiviral activity was highly specific to CMV. Although the drug could not destroy existing CMV in the body, it could stop viral replication and the invasion of healthy cells if it was used indefinitely.

By 1983, company researchers believed that ganciclovir curbed CMV retinitis. That fateful observation did not result in an approved drug for six more years. Depending on whom you ask, the saga of those lost years illustrates either the importance of restricting access to a drug until placebo-controlled trials are completed or the obstinacy of scientists and regulators unable to see the forest for the trees.

In early 1984, Syntex alerted the FDA to ganciclovir's promise and asked for permission to distribute it without charge until testing and marketing could get under way. At the time, no other drug was effective against CMV retinitis, and the FDA said yes. The company immediately began handing out the drug on a compassionate-use basis to any doctor who asked for it.

It soon became obvious to medical professionals and casual observers alike that ganciclovir worked. Therein lay the root of the ensuing problems.

Over the next three years Syntex handed out the drug to some 5,000 people at a cost to the company estimated at $25 million. Meanwhile, Burroughs Wellcome developed its own version of the drug, and the two companies battled for the rights to the ganciclovir patent—and thus the privilege of eventually selling it. While awaiting a decision from the U.S. Patent Office, BW also passed out ganciclovir, reaching another 1,300 people.

Syntex was granted the ganciclovir patent in March 1987, and BW dropped out of the picture. A few months later, Syntex asked the FDA to approve the drug, claiming that a traditional placebo-controlled trial was not only unnecessary, but was by then unethical because the drug's effectiveness was so obvious. A placebo trial was also unfeasible—neither doctors nor their patients had much interest in dummy pills. Not when the likely result was blindness and when the drug could be obtained by other means.

Syntex instead supported its application with data collected in four separate studies of participants who had obtained ganciclovir through the compassionate-use program. In doing so, the company flouted almost every existing standard of science. Its data was fragmented and difficult to interpret, and the forms used to track the compassionate use of the drug did not provide anything like the usual level of detail. Medical observations were irregular and incompletely recorded. Too many physicians had administered ganciclovir to assure uniformity; drug dosages and treatment regimens varied widely. The endpoints used to gauge the drug's effectiveness were poorly defined, and the controls that traditionally provide a basis of comparison were absent.

Moreover, most of the information had been retrospectively collected; in other words, researchers went back to original hospital records to learn what they could from patient charts, rather than monitoring patients as they took the drug. Syntex offered no data to support a particular dosage, no assurance that ganciclovir's benefits would outweigh its long-run side effects, and no way to assess how long treatment should last.

But Syntex's most egregious sin appeared to be its willingness to make ganciclovir available to everyone who needed it.

On October 26, 1987, an FDA advisory committee met to consider the Syntex application. Ellen Cooper set the tone of the meeting in her opening remarks. She criticized the ganciclovir data and said it fell far short of usual FDA requirements. "In some respects, what we are really left with is little better than a mass of anecdotal information," she said.

The scientific presentations that day confirmed her judgment. They were, according to Stephen Straus, a NIAID researcher and member of the advisory committee, "a perfect display of investigational anarchy," a classic example of how not to develop a drug. And yet, in a disturbing irony that would haunt committee members for some time to come, there was a clear consensus that ganciclovir was effective against CMV retinitis. John Mills, head of San Francisco General's Infectious Disease Department, called the evidence "close to overwhelming."

Then he lambasted everyone involved in the drug's development. "I think that the data that we saw today was terrible. And I think we are all to blame. I think the manufacturers are to blame; I think the Food and Drug Administration is to blame; and I think the investigators are to blame." Mills said that someone—anyone—should have stepped forward to declare that "we can't let this drug get away from us."

But by the time of the advisory committee meeting, it was too late. Ganciclovir had slipped through the cracks of the system. In a frantic effort to salvage it, one committee member proposed that ganciclovir be approved for first-phase use, in which a high dose of ganciclovir was injected intravenously for a brief period of time, but not for the second, indefinite phase, where a much lower dose was used. Based on the strength of the data, there was a certain abstract logic to his reasoning. But the practical implications were horrifying. "What you are actually suggesting is that we should use the drug to pull somebody out of the water, save somebody from drowning, but then drop him off again and let him drown," said Itzhak Brook, the committee's chairman. The suggestion was dismissed.

Instead, committee members decided not even to try the first rescue attempt. They would not vote their instincts. Gut feeling told them ganciclovir worked, but they lacked hard data to prove it. And so the committee said no to ganciclovir. There were just two dissenting votes—cast by the two ophthalmologists on the committee.

Based on established procedure, the FDA advisory committee was absolutely right—Syntex had not done the studies traditionally required to declare a drug effective. The problem, of course, was that the drug worked, and everyone knew it.

The committee's rejection of ganciclovir set off a cacophony of protest. "If a patient has CMV and doesn't get ganciclovir, he goes blind. If he gets ganciclovir, he doesn't go blind," said one ophthalmologist. "If ever there was clear-cut evidence that a drug worked, it was this." AIDS activists demanded that the decision be reconsidered. ACT UP fumed and threatened dire consequences. "We will agitate until it becomes impossible for advisory committees, whose members appear to have no knowledge or sympathy for those people who live with AIDS daily, to consign such drugs as ganciclovir to regulatory limbo," said an ACT UP spokesman. "This is a war as real as any. Give us the weapons so that we can defend ourselves."

But FDA Commissioner Frank Young defended the committee's decision with a comment that was echoed time and again by the medical establishment. "We can't accept testimonials," he said.

Tony Fauci, head of the National Institute of Allergy and Infectious Diseases, called the messy situation a vicious Catch-22: "Those of us who used the drug know it works, the data isn't sufficient to prove it works, you have to do a clinical trial, nobody wants to be on the clinical trial because they know the drug works." He grumbled about the resultant deadlock and said all the players were going around and around in circles without getting anywhere.

Ganciclovir remained available on a compassionate-use basis. But doctors treating patients terrified of going blind reminded the FDA that wasn't good enough because some private physicians and most hospital-based clinics were poorly equipped or unwilling to do the lengthy paperwork necessary to secure an unapproved drug. Once again, patients needed political clout, medical sophistication, or geographical proximity to get the drugs they needed.

Why did Syntex fail to design the type of study the FDA traditionally required? Rumor had it that the FDA had clearly suggested it would approve ganciclovir on the basis of the limited data available, since the drug was obviously effective. Many people felt Syntex was being punished because it had responded compassionately to patient pleas for the drug.

Calvin Kunin, an advisory committee member, felt that was a

simplistic view. He claimed the drug company would not have been so easily misled: "The pharmaceutical industry is not naïve. They can design a perfectly fine study if they want to. They obviously didn't want to."

One possible reason was the Syntex–Burroughs Wellcome patent dispute. Until Syntex knew for sure that it would win the intercompany battle, it was reluctant to invest in costly, full-scale clinical trials. Stephen Straus emphasized this point, telling the advisory committee: "I must think that the fact that there were two companies competing made it not financially worth their while to do an expensive study until they had the patent for this and the right to the development of the drug." There was also speculation that Syntex had tried to pull a fast one, fostering consumer pressure on the FDA so that it would buckle and approve ganciclovir without having to bother with expensive trials. The precedent-setting implications of that approach would obviously make the FDA leery.

Whatever actually went wrong, the FDA's message seemed clear enough: releasing a drug on a compassionate-use basis could compromise the company's chance to win marketing approval. The decision not to approve ganciclovir had a chilling effect. Fluconazole—manufactured by Pfizer and being tested as a treatment for cryptococcal meningitis—had been widely available while formal research studies continued. Suddenly it became hard to get.

For neither the first time nor the last, the patients and the drug companies were allied in their alarm over the government decision. "The FDA sent a very clear signal to the drug community and what it said is, 'Folks, don't do what Syntex did,'" said activist Jay Lipner. "It looked to us like they had taken a gigantic step backwards away from the availability of drugs."

At a time when the FDA was under tremendous pressure to expand access to unapproved drugs, the ganciclovir decision sent shivers of fear throughout the drug industry.

In tense summit conferences following the rejection of ganciclovir, representatives from Syntex and the FDA huddled to talk about the best way to generate the missing scientific information without using placebo controls—that is, without sacrificing the eyesight of half the trial participants on the altar of "clean" data.

A compromise design for a new trial was announced. The trial was to involve only patients with CMV on the periphery of the retina, where it did not yet affect sight. Under the plan, all participants would get an initial intensive dose of ganciclovir; afterward, they would be randomly assigned to receive either a placebo or a maintenance dose of the active drug. Both groups would be monitored continuously. At the first indication that infection was advancing toward the center of the retina, patients on placebo would be pulled from the study and given ganciclovir.

But there was a catch. Before committing itself to the trial, Syntex circulated the protocol to three ethics experts—and all three called it unethical. Given the weight of the evidence, they said, patients with CMV retinitis should under no circumstances be denied access to ganciclovir. The study was put on hold. Discussions continued, but no consensus was reached. Nine months dragged by.

In the summer of 1988, with the heat turned on from patients, regulators, and politicians, Syntex decided that maybe the rejected peripheral retinitis study was okay after all. The obvious question was, if that study was unethical nine months before, why was it acceptable now? Alternatively, if the study could actually pass muster, why had so much time been wasted before the trial was launched? No one had any answers.

Instead, federal officials rushed to praise the "new" study design, to be launched as ACTG Protocol 071. Daniel Hoth, who had been brought in from the National Cancer Institute to help run the ACTG system, called it a "state-of-the-art" trial. The FDA boasted that its willingness to approve the study design—which, after all, did not fit the strict definitions of a full-fledged placebo-controlled trial—demonstrated great flexibility. But many others declared that new trials were an absurd waste of money. "We didn't have 'clean data,' but we had so much evidence on it that there was not one clinician in this country who wasn't using ganciclovir for CMV retinitis," complained Jim Eigo. One New York physician called the study "mean," noting that CMV infection was erratic and that Protocol 071 might allow patients to lose a part of their sight before they became qualified for the drug.

Worse, the trial was coercive. In order to accrue patients, the FDA clamped down on easy access to ganciclovir, canceling the long-standing compassionate-use program. A much more limited Treatment

IND, open only to patients whose sight was imminently threatened by CMV retinitis, was substituted.

In theory, Protocol 071 was supposed to get under way at the same time that access to ganciclovir was curtailed. It didn't work out that way. Incredibly, red tape and a lack of urgency still prevailed. Just one of the forty-five centers participating in the trial was ready to enroll patients when the lid on compassionate use was nailed shut. Physician and patient rage boiled over. The FDA bowed to their pressure and agreed that Syntex could continue distributing ganciclovir to any patient not enrolled on Protocol 071. The drug once again became widely available. But it remained unapproved.

MOVING THE FDA OFF THE DIME

It took Tony Fauci's intervention to help change that situation.

Fauci had already begun to establish a rapport with AIDS activists. One Christmas he invited several leaders within the gay community to dinner at Jim Hill's house. Hill was NIAID's deputy director, who also happened to be an amateur gourmet chef and cooked an elaborate meal that night. Fauci spoke frankly as the men ate. He complained that many of his remarks had been taken out of context and that his good-faith efforts to explain the bureaucratic process had been deliberately thrown back in his face. Once, for example, he had mentioned casually that his agency could use some more office space. Shortly afterward, demonstrators appeared below his window carrying signs that read, "Fauci: Space isn't the answer, you're killing us."

"I think that is a cheap shot," he groused. "I was just trying to give you people a good feel for what is going on." He went on, "Do you really believe the things you put in the fliers? Do you really believe that this is a concerted effort on my part or the NIH's part to commit genocide or interfere with the effort of trying to get drugs out, or is that just your way of calling attention, to try and get people moving a little bit more quickly? Believe it or not, I'm one of the best friends you have."

By the end of the decade that friendship had evolved in curious ways. Eventually a surprising level of mutual respect developed in a relationship that also remained highly adversarial. Fauci established an especially close rapport with ACT UP New York, probably the highest-level federal official to have done so. He liked to joke that he was more accessible to activist representatives than to his own wife, Christine Grady, a nurse at the Institute.

Fauci had a special knack for taking barbs in stride. "I have been burned in effigy so many times it really doesn't matter," he said. "In fact, it has led to a very good relationship. They know that I still back them, that I'm still sensitive to them despite all those names that I have been called." He publicly praised the activists' knowledge of how the system works, and their persistence and success in applying "constructive pressure" on regulators and researchers.

They, in turn, felt they had found a well-placed ally. By the time of the 1990 International AIDS Conference in San Francisco—which some activists chose to boycott and others attended to boo and hiss many of the public officials who spoke—Tony Fauci got a standing ovation for his troubles.

His role in the ganciclovir saga was one of his most visible attempts to mediate between activists and the federal bureaucracy.

In January 1989, Fauci was in San Francisco to speak at an AIDS meeting being held at the St. Francis Hotel. Just before he stepped to the podium, ACT UP representatives popped up from the audience and began blowing whistles. Within minutes they had covered the hotel conference room with red tape. "You're killing us with red tape," they chanted for several minutes before dispersing.

With characteristic bemusement, Fauci complimented them on the careful organization of the demonstration. He knew the attention-getting device would not detract from the frank dialogue he had already had with the activists. Earlier that day, Fauci had met in his hotel room with several men with CMV retinitis who had described the human impact of ganciclovir's unapproved status. And he was obviously moved.

"We are in an untenable situation," one man told Fauci. "Somebody has got to break the vicious cycle. Will you help us?"

One of the people in the room that morning was Terry Sutton. By all accounts, Sutton was a remarkable young man. A teacher of emotionally disturbed teenagers in San Francisco until he was diagnosed with AIDS at the age of thirty-one, friends claimed Sutton found a spiritual strength after he became ill. His courage and determination in the face of tragedy helped light a fire beneath the advocacy movement in San Francisco.

Sutton's militancy grew with his commitment to political action. In the early years of the epidemic, when little was known about AIDS except the need to ease the process of dying, he volunteered at the Shanti Project, which provided hospice care and counseling to terminally ill patients. Later he decided that while compassion had its place, rage was more appropriate. In sync with an increasingly sophisticated political movement, Sutton organized "A Time to Shine," a benefit to bring people with AIDS to Washington to participate in the first national gay and lesbian demonstration.

At the San Francisco meeting with Fauci, Sutton made a strong case for getting ganciclovir approved. Then he put another issue on the table. Although it was considered safe, ganciclovir did have some disturbing side effects, including disorientation, the depletion of white blood cells, rashes, blood clots, and nausea. But ganciclovir's real problem, said Sutton, was that a significant portion of the AIDS population could not take it along with AZT because both had the dangerous side effect of suppressing the bone marrow.

That presented AIDS patients with a wrenching choice: surrender AZT and save their sight, or go blind in order to continue on the only antiviral medication available at the time. Almost everyone who thought hard about that decision opted for ganciclovir. One physician commented that "they would rather live for four months and be able to see than live for six months and go blind."

On his flight back to Washington, Fauci thought hard about what he had just heard. These men are right, he told himself. Something must be done.

Back in Bethesda, he looked again at the eyes of patients being treated at NIH clinics and knew that the drug worked. "One day the retinitis was there and a week later it was gone," said Fauci. He called investigators attempting to accrue patients into Protocol 071, the controversial peripheral retinitis study.

"How is the accrual going?" he asked.

"Patients aren't signing up," he was told.

A week later, Fauci made another round of telephone calls to the same investigators and asked the same question. Just one person had signed up in the last eight days. At that rate, Fauci calculated it would be 1998 before the trial was filled.

He arranged a meeting of his staff to confirm his suspicions. "It's my impression this drug works, is that correct?" he asked. Everyone agreed that it was.

Fauci began to agitate for the approval of ganciclovir, telephoning Frank Young to ask him to reconsider the value of all the anecdotal information that had already been collected. It was an audacious move, considering that drug approval was clearly the FDA's domain. But NIAID was moving more aggressively into AIDS drug research and Tony Fauci, it seemed, wanted to do the right thing.

"Look Frank, we have to re-look at the data," said Fauci.

Ganciclovir advocates had been saying the same thing for years. But from his vantage point within the federal bureaucracy, Fauci obviously commanded more attention. His conviction that the drug was a crucial weapon in the limited arsenal of AIDS therapies set the stage for the FDA's decision a few months later to approve the drug at last.

Five years after Syntex started handing out ganciclovir on a compassionate-use basis, and more than 1½ years after approval was first denied, the FDA's advisory committee met again to consider the drug. By then, ganciclovir had already been approved in eleven other countries.

The FDA seemed ready to back down; finally there was a consensus that ganciclovir had to be licensed. "What they did is stage this very elaborate charade in which essentially the same data, dressed up in new clothes, was presented before the advisory committee," claimed Jay Lipner. "And this time, magically, the advisory committee said, 'yes, we think this drug should be marketed.' "

Protocol 071 had enrolled fewer than twenty patients by the time the advisory committee met, and it had generated no information worthy of analysis. No other placebo-controlled trials had been conducted. The committee did have three additional studies to consider, but data from two of them—one conducted at San Francisco General Hospital and one in France—had not been supplied early enough for committee members to assess independently. The third study, presented by Douglas Jabs of Johns Hopkins Hospital, simply reviewed past patient experience, like its much-criticized predecessors.

In short, by traditional standards—the standards that had been so rigidly applied before—the data was as limited as ever. All the committee could conclude was that "these studies go in the right direction," a statement that could have been made many years earlier. Yet that day, by a vote of 8–0, with one abstention, the advisory committee recommended approval of ganciclovir.

"There was no change in the evidence from the disapproval to the approval," said Peter Barton Hutt. "There was a change in political climate." Six weeks later the FDA accepted the committee's recommendation and on June 27, 1989, ganciclovir became a fully licensed drug.

FURY OVER FOSCARNET

Meanwhile, foscarnet had begun to create a stir. Early trials suggested the antiviral drug was just as effective as ganciclovir in staving off CMV retinitis, and it was compatible with AZT.

The foscarnet story was in many ways inextricably linked to the story of Terry Sutton. Sutton had two requests that weren't hard to understand: he wanted to keep his eyesight and he wanted to live as long as possible. His medical tests indicated that he needed AZT. But in August 1988, doctors told him he had CMV retinitis. Faced with a no-win decision, Sutton abandoned AZT so that he could take ganciclovir in the hopes of staving off blindness. He should never have been put in that bind.

Astra Pharmaceutical Products held the patent on foscarnet. But the Swedish-based company would not allow anyone who had ever taken ganciclovir to participate in its trials. There was no scientific logic to this restriction; the body eliminates ganciclovir within twenty-four hours after it is ingested. Astra's real concern was satisfying FDA's demand for pure data. In order to get the most homogeneous patient population possible—and thus assure the agency that the drug under investigation, rather than some other factor, had produced a given result—researchers commonly impose blanket restrictions on the eligible subject population. It was simply easier to bar all people who had used ganciclovir than to justify exceptions.

That meant Terry Sutton could not enroll in a foscarnet trial. In one of the epidemic's many ironies, Sutton lived directly across the street from Davies Hospital, in the hills overlooking San Francisco's Castro District, where foscarnet trials were being conducted. But the sign hanging from Sutton's window—"Gosh darnit, I want my foscarnet"—brought him no attention from the researchers inside.

Fauci had promised to look further into the foscarnet problem, but Sutton wasn't about to sit on his hands in the interim. In early January 1989, he led a sit-in at San Francisco General Hospital, where the drug was also under study. The demonstrators blocked access to the pharmacy and began chanting, "Foscarnet is on our minds, we don't want to go blind." Then they banged on the pharmacy door and hollered, "We want foscarnet. We want foscarnet now."

From behind the door, a man called out, "Behave!"—an admonishment Sutton said he hadn't heard since he was a boy.

"Behave, be blind!" the protestors yelled back. Television viewers around the Bay Area that night watched the event replayed on the local news.

But the drama was modest compared to Sutton's next escapade that month—shutting down the Golden Gate Bridge. Some of his friends thought he was going too far, and warned against violence. The former teacher said he had no other options. "We have got to become someone's emergency," he declared.

The carefully plotted event took place during the height of the morning rush hour. The bridge was shrouded in fog as the protestors began chanting and blocking traffic. Within a few minutes, cars were backed up all the way into Marin County. Motorists honked in fury but they could not drown out the angry shouts: "Forty-eight thousand dead from AIDS, where is George?" and "AIDS is genocide." Sutton was dragged off to jail that morning, and the story leapt on to front-page headlines.

Sutton was running a fever of 104 when he was released from jail soon afterward. It was the beginning of the end. His health deteriorated steadily after the Golden Gate Bridge blow-out, and by March he was hospitalized. As he lay in his hospital bed hovering on the brink of delirium, his doctors offered him the opportunity he had been pleading for—the chance to take foscarnet.

But the system hadn't changed. Rather, an exception had been made for Sutton, who asked indignantly, "Are they trying to buy me off? Do they think they can silence me?" He told his doctor he would not take foscarnet unless the drug was made available to everyone who needed it.

His sister begged him to change his mind, arguing that he'd be more valuable alive, and challenging the system, than being martyred for the cause. Sutton held fast to his position for one long day and night. By the following morning he had lost the opportunity to rethink his logic. That day he lapsed into a final illness. He was in a coma for most of his remaining hours, but at the very end, he was awake and clearly panicked, biting his tongue and grinding his teeth as seizure followed terrifying seizure.

Early on the morning of April 11, 1989, Terry Sutton died.

A few days later his ashes were scattered at sea. As the boat sailed past the Golden Gate Bridge, where Sutton had made his final stand, the mourners tossed roses into the steel-blue waters of San Francisco Bay and released dozens of balloons carrying ACT UP's unequivocal message: "Silence = Death."

A few weeks later, several hundred demonstrators shut down traffic at Market and Castro streets, chanting, "Who killed Terry Sutton?" Clearly, private industry and public health officials shared some of the guilt.

In part because of the publicity surrounding Sutton's life and death, the number of approved clinical trials for foscarnet was gradually increased and eligibility criteria were loosened. But Astra still refused to apply for a Treatment IND, claiming uncertainty about the drug's safety. Some thought the ganciclovir debacle was the real source of Astra's timidity.

ACT UP wrote the Swedish Consulate a letter, asking them to pressure Astra for pre-approval release. "People can get foscarnet on compassionate use in many European countries. Then why not here? Any why not now, before we lose another life, before another friend goes blind?"

The FDA signed on with the forces of discontent. Weary of waiting for a corporate initiative, the agency actively encouraged Astra to apply for a Treatment IND and told the company just how to structure its application. That proactive stance was a far cry from the passive role the FDA had taken in reviewing ganciclovir.

But Astra continued to resist, and access to the drug languished. ACT UP staged a "zap," the tried-and-true technique that involves besieging a target—most often corporate or government officials suspected of holding up progress on a drug—with a barrage of telephone calls and faxes. Hundreds of calls went to top management, including Lars Bildman, Astra's chief executive officer, but the company wouldn't budge.

On September 21, 1990, Astra finally submitted its application for drug approval to the FDA. Only then did it announce that foscarnet would be available on a compassionate-use basis to patients who had failed ganciclovir or were intolerant of the drug. But the eligibility criteria were strict, and not everyone who wanted foscarnet could get it. Physicians who asked for the drug initially had to complete a seventy-six-page case report form for each patient, a ludicrous demand.

Astra made it especially difficult to get the drug on an ongoing, maintenance basis. It was just as Itzhak Brook, the chairman of the ganciclovir advisory committee, had warned three years earlier when that drug was being considered for approval: patients were being thrown life preservers, then left floundering helplessly after they were snatched away. That remained the situation for a full year, until the FDA approved foscarnet on September 27, 1991. Even then, its $21,000-a-year price tag meant that many patients would be unable to afford the sight-saving drug.

The ganciclovir/foscarnet mess had one significant benefit: it helped clarify an idea in Tony Fauci's mind. Syntex's failure, he thought, had not been its decision to expand access to ganciclovir, but the fact that it did not simultaneously conduct a formal trial. Astra's bungle was just the reverse—not its insistence on carefully controlled trials, but its refusal to loosen access to foscarnet at the same time.

A mechanism should be developed so that such disasters do not happen again, thought Fauci, who was especially moved by Terry Sutton's vexing plight. Jay Lipner's fears that the FDA's ganciclovir decision would eviscerate the concept of expanded access were soon laid to rest. Two months after Sutton's death, Tony Fauci proposed a new tool for providing early access to AIDS drugs.

14

PARALLEL TRACK AND THE PROMISE OF DDI

THE FIRST STORMY DECADE of AIDS was drawing to a close when some real signs of change became apparent. There were hints that the federal bureaucracy was at last growing more responsive. Although President Bush was still virtually ignoring the epidemic, the FDA had been sobered by its experience with ganciclovir and finally began to take a more innovative approach to evaluating new drugs, and Tony Fauci continued to win respect from patient advocates. Martin Delaney, head of Project Inform, spoke with conciliatory words: "Regulators today understand that we activists are not proponents of quackery or free-market theorists set upon the dissolution of drug regulation. We, for our part, recognize that Drs. Fauci and Young are not murderous war criminals presiding over the deliberate destruction of people with AIDS." To anyone familiar with the years of bitterness that preceded that comment, Delaney sounded like a changed man.

There was still a long road to travel before promising research was likely to pay off. There were grave concerns about the design of drug trials, and ethical qualms about a system that allowed white gay men to get experimental drugs much more readily than women or minorities, especially drug users.

But the terrain was clearly changing as activist voices began to be heard in Washington's corridors of power. Some said the honeymoon began with the enthusiasm about parallel track and the promise of ddI.

FAUCI'S PROPOSAL

In March 1989, Fauci traveled to New York with Peggy Hamburg, his top assistant, intent on meeting ACT UP on its home ground. He thought it was time to improve the channels of communication. In his capacity as NIAID director, Tony Fauci was in charge of the government's entire AIDS clinical research effort, and it wasn't working very well.

At his spring meeting, Fauci listened closely to the litany of complaints about the ACTG system. The activists, as usual, were well informed, and alerted him to the depth of patient resentment over the design and pacing of drug trials. Fauci was especially disturbed by their obvious bitterness, recognizing that if patients felt investigators were insensitive to their needs, they would not feel obliged to comply with study requirements. That meant the traditional scientific process was heading for a breakdown.

The session convinced Fauci of two things: as it was being applied, Treatment IND hadn't proved to be effective enough in expanding patient access to experimental drugs, and activists had to be given a more vocal role in shaping the research effort. Soon afterward, Fauci became more outspoken, and more public, in his criticisms of the Treatment IND program. Then he began to advocate an alternative.

At the June 1989 AIDS conference in Montreal, Fauci took a "walk in the woods" with Larry Kramer. The "woods," in this case, were the streets of the French Canadian city, where they strolled late one evening. The resulting detente was dramatic, a historic rapprochement that echoed the breakthrough achieved by arms control negotiator Paul Nitze and his Soviet counterpart during another walk in the woods five years before.

A year before he bumped into Fauci in Montreal, Kramer had written an open letter, which had been published in the *Village Voice* and the *San Francisco Examiner*, calling the NIAID's top man "an incompetent idiot," and the ACTG system he ran "a system of waste, chaos and uselessness." The two hadn't talked since, but Fauci greeted Kramer warmly, apparently willing to let bygones be bygones. Fauci was focused more on a new idea than on an old grudge, and he wanted to tell Kramer all about it.

As the men walked together through the streets of Montreal,

Kramer learned that Fauci intended to endorse a concept called "parallel track." The idea had been germinating for months on both coasts. Jim Eigo and Martin Delaney had discussed it together, and Eigo had broached it publicly in January. Now Fauci was about to give parallel track an official stamp of approval.

His formal announcement came in San Francisco at the end of June, where he had gone to address a medical forum during the city's Treatment Awareness Week, organized primarily by Project Inform. The concept was that patients who could not join a study—because they did not meet strict eligibility criteria, because the study was full, or because they lived too far away—could get promising experimental drugs anyway. One set of patients would receive the drug from their personal physicians if they did not qualify for the formal scientific studies. At the same time, the more closely monitored clinical trials—typically comprising persons with a fairly homogeneous medical profile—would move forward.

"I thought we could kill two birds with one stone—the two birds were compliance with the clinical trial and sensitivity to people who have no options," Fauci explained.

Fauci knew there were risks to parallel track—beginning with almost certain resistance from staunch traditionalists within the ACTG system. Still, he said, "the government ought not force patients into formal trials by holding a gun to their heads. We have got to rethink the rigidity with which we exclude people."

With his San Francisco announcement, Fauci became a hero to the activist community. Jim Eigo praised his foresight, commenting, "The AIDS establishment has to realize that unless it secures the goodwill of the communities affected by AIDS, those trials will never get done. The establishment's embrace of parallel track would be a demonstrable gesture toward securing that goodwill."

Much work remained to be done. First of all, Fauci's San Francisco parallel-track announcement had taken his colleagues by surprise. Some political fences needed mending. And Fauci had made only a bare-bones announcement; others were going to have to flesh out the concept, which put the FDA in an awkward position. As the nation's drug regulator, the agency would have to set up guidelines for a concept it had not initiated, had not endorsed, and did not believe was necessary.

The relationship between the FDA and NIAID had been a troubled one for a long time. Now, simmering resentments threatened to boil over.

Ellen Cooper, like most others at the FDA, had no advance warning about Fauci's speech; she read it the following day in the newspapers. She was startled and resentful to see the initiative for expanded access snatched from her agency's hands. As far as she and others at the FDA were concerned, Treatment IND could have accomplished essentially the same goals.

"You don't need a new entity called parallel track," said Cooper later. In fact, just weeks before the "San Francisco Surprise," she and other FDA officials had met with activists to talk about ways to get ddI, a drug closely related to AZT, to patients before the drug was approved. But now it was NIAID, and not the FDA, that was basking in the limelight.

Fauci claimed that politics wasn't a factor in his decision to propose the parallel-track initiative. "I was trying to preserve the integrity of the clinical trial process," he said. "If you are trying to do a clinical trial in a population that does not believe that you are sensitive to their needs, you will be unsuccessful. My motivations were 100 percent for the clinical trial process."

Almost surely, though, there was more to the picture—politics has something to do with almost everything in Washington. More specifically, Fauci and Frank Young each had political hay to make by gaining the support of the AIDS community.

Young was in an especially delicate position. Treatment IND was the cornerstone of the FDA's recent AIDS drug policy innovations, and the commissioner did not want that hard-fought effort dismissed. Nor did he want Tony Fauci, who had a lot to gain by seeing his concept implemented, stealing too much thunder. Young, according to one activist, was "tired of being out-Faucied."

But he was also politically embattled. A scandal over generic drugs had burst into the headlines, and Frank Young looked bad. Several FDA employees had been accused of accepting bribes from sponsors to speed drug approval. At congressional hearings a year after the scandal broke, the extent of the corruption came to light: more than one-third of all generic drugs sold in the United States were controlled by firms that had paid off FDA employees or secured drug approval fraudulently. No one accused Young personally of improper behavior, but everyone knew it had happened on his watch.

Within a few months, the generic drug scandal cost Frank Young his job. It would be well over a year before his replacement was found. While he still clung to his post, the commissioner was eager to demonstrate the agency's flexibility. It wasn't going to be easy for him to dismiss parallel track.

When Henry Waxman hit the gavel to open congressional hearings on parallel track in July, some 7,000 people were enrolled in ACTG trials, a small fraction of the million estimated to be infected with HIV. "Most can just read about drugs they cannot get," said Waxman. "We have lived with a policy of limited distribution today so that we will have adequate information for tomorrow." Increasingly, that policy seemed inadequate.

Frank Young suggested that Treatment IND be repolished, not replaced altogether. Jim Eigo declared that because of its narrow application, Treatment IND was discredited within the gay community. In attacking efforts to breathe new life into it, Eigo turned to Young at the Waxman hearings and made his point by a colorful mixing of metaphors: "Forgive me, Commissioner Young, but given the failed history of the program, I have no reason to believe that this year's model is anything more than the same old lemon with tail fins. And I tell you, the baby won't fly, and I'm afraid it will be next year till we find out, and the year after that till FDA gets around to retinkering with what we already know doesn't work. With AIDS we just don't have the time."

James Mason, head of the Public Health Service, which had both FDA and NIAID under its wing, was said to be irritated that Fauci had proposed parallel track without consulting his higher-ups. But apparently he was even more perturbed by the split between the two agencies, which made the PHS appear to be at war with itself. In an effort to end the internecine bickering, Mason stamped parallel track with the Bush Administration's seal of approval.

Jay Lipner viewed Mason's endorsement as an attempt to restore peace to the family. Lipner said, "I think someone in the White House and at Health and Human Services finally woke up and said, "Hey, the guys are fighting in public. Young and Fauci are going after each other. This has to be resolved.' " Mason decreed, in effect, that the Public Health Service was to speak with one voice.

Another big obstacle had yet to be overcome: ACTG researchers had to line up behind parallel track. That proved difficult to arrange. Some of the ACTG researchers were furious at Fauci. In public, they tried to discredit parallel track by claiming it would undermine good science. Several investigators deliberately leaked word to the press that the new approach to expanding drug access might weaken enrollment in formal clinical trials.

In hushed whispers, and behind closed doors, the talk was also about parallel track's impact on their own careers. Their real fear was that the program would so debilitate traditional research that it could lead to the demise of the whole ACTG system.

DDI ENTERS THE PICTURE

Excitement about ddI informed discussions about parallel track.

Like AZT, ddI was one of "Broder's babies." Sam Broder and Hiroaki Mitsuya, the virologist who had played such a central role in AZT's development, had long suspected the drug held promise because it was also a nucleoside analogue that inhibits the reverse transcriptase enzyme and a close chemical cousin of AZT. Mitsuya had first spotted ddI back in 1985 when he was scouring chemical reagent catalogs, looking for other drugs in the same family.

Like AZT, ddI prevents the AIDS virus from copying its genetic material. Scientists don't know whether it is superior to AZT, but its longer half-life means it does not have to be administered as frequently. It is also uncertain whether ddI has more staying power than AZT, which typically loses effectiveness after a year or two. A more established fact is that the two drugs have differing side effects. The belief that ddI would prove less toxic led to the nickname "AZT without tears." Unlike AZT, ddI does not suppress bone marrow, but it is associated with peripheral neuropathy, a painful nerve problem in the hands and feet, and pancreatitis, an inflammation of the pancreas that can be fatal. A combination of the two therapies seems promising, since ddI may be effective against HIV strains that become insensitive to AZT. The hope, too, is that alternating the therapies will lessen their toxicities.

As ddI's commercial potential became more apparent, Broder showed he had learned a lesson from Burroughs Wellcome's ap-

proach to AZT, and did not intend to get burned again. In a gesture
as much symbolic as practical, Broder, Mitsuya, and Robert Yarchoan, an NCI colleague, all put their names on government patents
for ddI. That meant the scientists were entitled to a small share of
future royalties from the sale of the drug. But the crucial incentive
was to avoid a repeat of the AZT scandal. Broder wanted to make it
clear from the outset that government researchers had been involved
in ddI's development—and that, ethically and legally, they retained
a degree of control over its marketing.

As patent owner, NCI could designate the company that would get
the license to test and develop ddI and it sought out Bristol-Myers,
one of the nation's Big Ten pharmaceutical firms, for the job. In
negotiations, conducted with assistance from the U.S. Department of
Commerce, Broder exercised his leverage by inserting a "reasonable
price clause" in NCI's licensing contract with Bristol-Myers. "This is
a free enterprise country, and companies are entitled to profits and
returns on their investments," said Broder. "But the government has
a legitimate interest in the final price of a product, not only because
government research is involved but because the government is a
major customer for drugs. From the patient's point of view, if you
can't afford a drug or don't have access to it, for you the drug was
never invented."

Under the "reasonable price clause," Bristol-Myers had to price
ddI fairly, although that term was not defined and it was uncertain
who would enforce it. Still, it gave the federal government a defensi-
ble right to revoke the company's exclusive marketing rights if it tried
to charge too much for ddI.

At the Montreal AIDS conference, Sam Broder had talked enthusiastically about the drug's potential, and in his San Francisco speech,
Fauci suggested the drug was a natural prototype for testing parallel
track. In July 1989, several months after the one hundred thousandth
case of AIDS in the United States had been recorded, Broder published promising results from his Phase I ddI study. As Phase II trials
were being developed, a familiar scenario began to unfold. Rumors
about the drug circulated on the AIDS underground, and the buyers'
clubs began prowling for bootleg sources of ddI. Soon the Healing
Alternatives Foundation in San Francisco found a Canadian source

willing to ship the drug across the border. By summer the goods began to arrive.

Tony Fauci, Ellen Cooper, and the AIDS activists did not want the old story replayed. Instead of allowing the drug to slip out of their control, they began a remarkably unified attempt to persuade Bristol-Myers to distribute free ddI to patients who didn't qualify for formal trials.

The company had no legal obligation to release the drug early. Its decision to do so was calculated, risky, and shrewd. It was also a significant departure from a corporate tradition of caution. The initial costs of manufacturing and distributing an unapproved drug were certain to be substantial. Worse, if the drug proved toxic, Bristol-Myers could be liable, and future clinical trials would almost surely be endangered.

On the other hand, if ddI proved safe and effective, most of the costly marketing work would already have been done. Physicians would be in the habit of using the drug, and the company would benefit from all the advance publicity. Bristol-Myers could also reasonably expect that by its compassionate response to patient needs, it was currying favor with the FDA and increasing the odds for swift approval if the data looked good.

Bristol-Myers eventually agreed to release ddI on an expanded-access basis. Rumor had it that the green light came directly from Richard Gelb, the company's CEO.

Larry Kramer was ecstatic over Bristol-Myers's decision and publicly praised the company for putting "compassion before greed." But a lot of particulars remained to be ironed out. The big unknown was just who would get ddI outside the trials.

August 17, 1989, was another busy day in the AIDS world.

At the Hyatt Regency Hotel in Bethesda, an FDA advisory committee was meeting to provide a sounding board for the parallel-track debate and to talk about exactly how it might work. The same day, the results of Protocol 019, showing that AZT could slow progression to AIDS, were being announced at a press conference in downtown Washington.

The activists were also making their voices heard that historic summer day. A hunger strike, which had started in Los Angeles and spread nationwide, was launched in Washington that morning. Participants said they would starve themselves to death unless parallel track was launched—a threat they fortunately did not carry out.

In a remarkable display of unity, seventeen different AIDS service and advocacy organizations had written a statement on parallel track and released it to the press that August morning. In their consensus statement, the group endorsed parallel track as the best hope "to address some of the most urgent problems posed by the AIDS epidemic: the rapidly expanding caseload, the proliferation of new promising treatments, the inability of traditional research institutions to test each promising therapy, the inability of most HIV-infected Americans to enroll in controlled clinical trials, and the use by many patients, out of necessity or choice, of other medications."

Valuable for the guidelines it proposed, the document was even more significant for the consensus it represented. Never before had the nation's leading AIDS activists managed to speak with one voice. Later they would parlay that new-found unity into other causes.

The hotel where the FDA advisory committee on parallel track was meeting was cool and comfortable. Which was just as well—dozens of speakers stepped to the podium and heated the room with their remarks. Activists in the audience upped the ante by standing against the meeting-room walls holding handmade signs that read, "The Faster You Act, the Longer We Live," and "Clocks Tick, People Die."

Many of the key players in the AIDS world had traveled to the Hyatt to have their say. James Mason put in a cameo appearance, and Tony Fauci and Frank Young stayed most of the day. The FDA, NIAID, and NIAID's parent agency, the National Institutes of Health, were represented by other highly placed officials as well. So was the Centers for Disease Control, which tracked the incidence of AIDS by race, sex, and risk group and kept the grim death tally. There were speakers from private industry, from university campuses, and from the patient advocacy community. Jeff Levi of the National Gay and Lesbian Task Force, who had made some enemies when he challenged the wisdom of Treatment IND, was there, and it was clear that he had come a long way in his thinking.

ACT UP brought a familiar cast of characters; New Yorkers Jim Eigo and Mark Harrington both spoke. So did Michelle Roland, an activist and medical student in California whose friend, Terry Sutton, had served as a painful illustration of the flaws in existing compassion-ate-use programs. Martin Delaney, representing Project Inform, and Don Abrams, from San Francisco General Hospital, also flew in from the West Coast. And Derek Hodel of the PWA Health Group came from New York to talk about the desperation for drugs that was driving patients underground.

In all, more than fifty presentations were made. The debate focused on whether a parallel track was needed at all—most speakers argued that it could reach more people than Treatment IND had been able to—and how best to design a viable program. The latter was the sticking point.

The questions raised that day had a familiar ring. How safe and effective did experimental therapies have to be before they were widely dispensed? Which drugs should be selected first for parallel track? Who would get access to unapproved drugs? Should they be available only for the sickest patients or the healthiest ones? How could equitable access be ensured for minority populations? How could the legitimacy of clinical trials be preserved if drugs were made available outside a trial setting? How would patient recruitment into formal trials be affected? What could be done to secure research data from drugs used in uncontrolled settings?

A man named Angelo Lau instilled a sense of urgency in the day's agenda when he described his plight to the committee in tragic detail. For a year, Lau had thrived on AZT, then seen his CD4 cell count plunge by 50 percent, a warning signal of infections to follow. AZT was not working for him anymore, and he was looking urgently for an antiviral alternative before his immune system collapsed. His di-lemma was not unusual; he was still too healthy to qualify for existing studies. Researchers told him he would have to get sicker before he could get a new drug.

Angelo Lau was afraid that later would be too late. "I have no objection to clinical trials," he said. "If there is one in which I would fit in, I would be very glad to go into it, but I cannot fit into them. I do not want to die and I do not have any other alternatives."

Tony Fauci defended increased accessibility to unproven drugs as "perfectly compatible" with good science and the mission of the National Institutes of Health while Jim Eigo went a step further, claiming that a trial with a parallel track would actually generate cleaner data. "If the people who are enrolled in the trial are desperate to get a drug at any cost, they will lie to get in and cheat while on protocol," he said. By contrast, Eigo believed that if a drug was available outside the trial to those who needed it, enrollees would more likely be "those who can abide by the trial's rigor."

Mindful that desperate patients might be moved to desperate measures, Martin Delaney warned that drugs had to be released cautiously. Anything less could sink the whole parallel-track concept, he said. "We are not talking about a crapshoot here. We are not inviting the floodgates to open and suddenly release every drug that somehow or other scrapes its way through Phase I."

At the same time, Delaney urged the committee to broaden its notion of risk. "When we talk about risks, we have to balance whatever risks we are taking by going forward in parallel track against the risk that we have already tacitly accepted here . . . the risk of doing nothing."

The committee also deliberated that day about how much data to gather on parallel-track drugs. Calvin Kunin, a committee member, warned against repeating the ganciclovir fiasco in which everyone got the drug on an expanded-access basis and good data never became available.

Still, most speakers emphasized that the first priority of parallel track was to provide treatment unavailable through other means, not to collect mountains of data. "The more paperwork we put out there in the community for doctors, the less cooperation we are going to get," said Delaney.

On the subject of data collection, at least, compromise was relatively easy and Jim Eigo was the voice of wisdom. He said that while data collection "should not drive the beast" of parallel track, "we would be fools" not to collect some of the information generated when an experimental drug was widely distributed.

There was less agreement as to whether drug companies would voluntarily distribute their drugs through parallel track, something few had done with Treatment IND. "How do we inspire them, motivate them, force them, convince them, cajole them to participate in this process?" asked Jeff Levi. One proposed solution was to link final marketing approval to a firm's willingness to supply drugs on parallel track.

Toward the end of the day, Mark Harrington called for aggressive government intervention to move parallel track forward. "Are we not in a war?" he asked. "If we were fighting a foreign enemy, the government would be issuing massive contracts and compelling large manufacturers to provide material. In the war on AIDS, new treatments are war material."

Jean McGuire, of the AIDS Action Council, also called for strong action. "We need to be radical and we need to be aggressive," she said.

But some in the audience thought the tenor of the debate was neither.

By early afternoon, Tom Lorango of ACT UP New York had enough. During the session devoted to public comment he rose to express his shock at the absence of urgency he sensed. "I cannot expect that you can understand the living hell that having HIV infection is," he said. "All I can ask is that you move as quickly and as effectively as possible, that you stop this endless haggling over minor points and get to the real issue, which is saving lives."

Lorango was not the only speaker to vent his rage. Larry Kramer did not hold back either, threatening dire consequences if parallel track was not implemented by the end of September. "If we do not get these drugs, you will see an uprising the likes of which you have never seen before since the Vietnam War in this country. We will sabotage all of your Phase II studies. We will continue to get our drugs on the underground. Our chemists will duplicate your formulas," he warned. Then Kramer suggested the committee remember the lessons of past uprisings. "Revolutions do not occur when there is no hope. Revolutions occur when there is hope and the system cannot keep up with the rising expectations of the maligned and the downtrodden and the discriminated against and the forgotten. And for ten years you have forgotten us. Starting today, I beg of you, I threaten you, make fucking history!"

Kramer didn't get parallel track by September. The final hour of the day's debate turned sour as participants disagreed on where to go next. A member of the audience accused the committee of "pissing away a whole fucking day." Someone else interrupted the proceed-

ings by chanting "two deaths an hour." Activists sitting in the audience dangled their wristwatches and shouted that time was being
wasted.

Several speakers pressed the committee to make specific recommendations to the FDA on a design for parallel track that very afternoon. But no bureaucratic decision had ever been made with such
haste, and the committee quickly nixed that suggestion.

Jean McGuire then suggested forming a small working group to
grapple with the many unresolved issues and to plan for the program's implementation. James Allen, director of the Public Health
Service's National AIDS Program Office, which was supposed to assemble the nuts and bolts of parallel track, pledged to move quickly
and he was as good as his word. The first meeting of the parallel-track
working group was held before the month's end.

At about the same time, Allen's office called a meeting in Washington
to discuss guidelines for handing out ddI outside ongoing trials. Some
said it went a bit overboard in its laudable efforts to obtain input.
"They invited everyone in the world," said Jay Lipner, who was
heavily involved in the push for expanded access to the drug. "Four
patient advocates, four community doctors, four researchers, four
representatives from the FDA, four from the NIH, four from Bristol-
Myers."

Although inclusiveness was always an activist goal, that first meeting was steeped more in politics than in medicine. No consensus was
reached, but it was an eye-opener for Bristol-Myers. "I'm not sure
they fully understood what they were getting into," Lipner recalled.
"At that meeting, the people from Bristol-Myers just sat there like the
four Smith Brothers, like the cough drops. They didn't say a word."
Lipner believed their silence stemmed from the startled recognition
of just how far they had agreed to stick out their necks.

Frustrated by the political climate in which the discussion was
shrouded, Lipner told the group about a meeting planned in New
York the next evening with community doctors interested in ddI.
Ellen Cooper was going to be there, and Lipner asked if a Bristol-
Myers representative would like to attend. The company agreed
enthusiastically. Fauci asked for an invitation, too, although he ended
up sending Peggy Hamburg as his emissary.

The very next night, Cooper, Hamburg, Eigo, and several Bristol-Myers representatives descended on Lipner's law office. Ten local physicians were there as well. Lipner recalled that the New York meeting "was all doctor talk, no politics," and, for that reason, proved a lot more productive. Doctors talked very specifically about what happened to patients who couldn't tolerate AZT and why alternatives were needed. The Bristol-Myers representatives took copious notes.

Predictably, Cooper asked for strict limitations on who would get expanded access to ddI. The activists, by contrast, wanted everyone to be allowed the drug. Eventually a middle ground was reached: ddI would be available on early release to those "with no other options."

In the weeks following the New York meeting, final agreement had to be reached on what constituted "no other options." Then there was some wrangling over appropriate dosage levels. Eleventh-hour reports about unexpectedly toxic drug side effects caused further delays. Grumblings among ACTG researchers, who circulated a private letter damning the whole concept of expanded access to ddI, also threatened to derail the efforts.

But in September, long before the formal parallel-track regulations were proposed, a two-tier system for distributing ddI was announced. Three ACTG Phase II trials, with total target enrollments of 2,600 patients, were planned. Two of them would compare ddI to AZT, while the third—the only one open to patients who could not tolerate AZT—studied ddI at three different doses. At the same time, the FDA said that anyone who was ineligible for the ACTG ddI trials could get the experimental drug if they had adverse reactions to AZT or continued to get sicker in spite of it.

As a result, there was broad access to ddI while rigorous research moved ahead. An unusual confluence of interests had made that possible. Bristol-Myers, conveniently, was a willing pioneer that recognized the link between good public relations and a sound business decision. Fauci was pleased to have concrete proof that parallel track was viable, while Young could cite ddI as an example of the FDA's flexibility, gaining good press when he needed it badly. Patients got the alternative to AZT they wanted and activists had tangible results to show from their increasing political clout.

For once, federal AIDS drug policy was developed more in a spirit of cooperation than strife. Parallel track had been launched.

15

RESEARCH ON TRIAL

The Limits of the Government System

Your choices were bewilderingly many; theories
about cause and cure were disorganized. The world
was waiting for someone to forge a clear path through
a forest of entangled images.

—MARK CALDWELL,
*The Last Crusade: The War
on Consumption*

THE AGENDA OF THE AIDS ACTIVISTS gradually shifted further from the
FDA. The agency's support for expanded access to ddI spoke volumes
about its new flexibility and a consensus slowly emerged among the
activists that the FDA had been pushed as far as it could go, at least
for the moment. No one, after all, wanted an anything-goes atmosphere to permeate either the drug industry or the agency that was
supposed to regulate it.

But drugs still weren't weaving through the testing labyrinths—
those operated at government-sponsored AIDS Clinical Trial Group
sites or elsewhere—fast enough. "Everyone is still acting as if they're
dealing with a slow-acting cancer," said Larry Kramer in despair.

Barry Gingell, the former director of medical information at GMHC, offered a sobering reminder of the human consequences of that pace as he described the downward spiral of a typical patient:

> The patient is usually jogging five to eight miles a day; he is usually working out at the gym two or three times a week, because he is afraid that he has been infected with the AIDS virus. And then one day while dressing he looks down at his thigh and he sees this purple bump, and he knows that indeed he has got Kaposi's sarcoma, and he comes in and we take a biopsy, and he waits a week to find out what it really is. He knows, and I know, and you know. But he waits through that limbo of a week to find out if he's going to be dead in five years, or not.
>
> And he comes in, and we tell him he has AIDS. And then slowly, inexorably, over the next two or three years, that young man has to watch himself daily, in the mirror, lose weight, become ashen, turn gray. He sees that body that was young and virile and handsome just a year ago, now become a shell.

By the end of 1991, more than $420 million had been sunk into the ACTG program yet it had not produced a single breakthrough drug. Despite its laudable intentions, NIAID's clinical trial system largely failed to rise above the bureaucratic mire. Researchers and patients had reached a standoff. In growing numbers, people with AIDS were refusing to enroll in clinical trials whose designs they disliked. Bitterness lingered over placebo-controlled trials and cheating was commonplace. Many people with AIDS were experimenting with such a wide range of approved and unapproved medications that it had become very hard to evaluate the effectiveness of a single drug. Community doctors, especially in rural areas that had not been overwhelmed by AIDS, often remained dangerously unaware of current research because of the long lag between a trial's completion and the publication of results.

And the White House leadership remained, as always, asleep at the wheel.

Clinical trials—how they are designed, who is allowed to participate in them, and what drugs get tested—were next to spark activist passions. NIAID bore the brunt of the criticism partly because it was

the largest single purveyor of AIDS research and partly because
activists felt they had more leverage over public institutions than over
profit-making pharmaceutical firms.

NIAID's RESEARCH VENTURE

To understand what went wrong requires a look back to the founding
of NIAID's clinical trials program. It was 1986, five years after the
epidemic was officially recognized, and more than a year after Congress had set aside the necessary funds. Borrowing the approach used
in cancer research, NIAID initially set up fourteen AIDS research
units at major academic and medical institutions around the country.
In response to a congressional demand, the research response to
AIDS was intensified with the addition of five more sites.

Institutions awarded the funds mostly had a long history of prestigious research and close ties to the medical establishment. They included some of America's most elite institutions: Stanford, UCLA,
Harvard, Johns Hopkins, Sloan-Kettering, the University of Miami,
and Duke University. Despite the demographics of the epidemic, no
research was based in the impoverished minority communities of
Harlem or the South Bronx; nor were there testing sites in the drug-
ravaged neighborhoods of Oakland, Liberty Hill, or East Los Angeles.
Patient advocates grumbled about discrimination and the inequities
of the system, but it would have been startling if things had turned
out any other way. After an unconscionable delay—some 30,000 people already had AIDS by then, and almost two-thirds of them were
dead—the biomedical establishment was finally mobilizing its attack.
Having been entrusted with millions of taxpayer dollars, government
officials felt obliged to turn to well-established research centers with
proven track records to run its clinical trials.

Fauci predicted that the research sites, originally called AIDS
Treatment Evaluation Units, would enroll 1,000 patients in trials in
their first six months of operation. AZT, foscarnet, HPA-23, ribavirin,
ddI, ddC, and alpha interferon were at the head of the testing lineup.
Once those tests got off the ground, he planned to launch a series of
small-scale, swift trials for other promising agents. Fauci's strategy
was devised on the assumption that an effective antiviral therapy
could be found, but he was not expecting quick results.

Then Burroughs Wellcome's Phase II AZT study proved successful. AIDS drug research changed dramatically at that point. The unexpected discovery of a drug that curbed HIV replication sent a shock wave through the scientific community. Rather than dissipate scarce resources on speculative agents, NIAID quickly reordered its research priorities, shelving virtually all the other tests it had planned. A slew of trials to assemble a fuller picture of AZT was substituted.

Enrollment problems began almost at once. In the first ten months, a meager 350 patients signed up for the trial, barely more than one-third of the number planned. For the most part, people with AIDS felt so alienated by the structure and design of the studies that they simply refused to participate.

Part of the problem was that, unlike the National Cancer Institute, NIAID had no trial system in place. A new infrastructure had to be created, staff had to be hired and trained, new facilities needed to be built and investigational standards had to be developed. Each step was time-consuming and costly. "It was like reinventing the wheel," said Mathilde Krim, who was closely monitoring the pace of research. "NIAID didn't have the facilities or the money to do it. NCI could have done it better and faster."

NIAID's staffing, resources, and political clout lagged behind its ambitious vision. The agency didn't even have the authority to reno- vate its own space, buy furniture, or hire top personnel without permission from higher-ups within the National Institutes of Health establishment. And rumor had it that Tony Fauci had been threatened with loss of his job by high-level White House officials if he complained too much about resource shortfalls. Small surprise, then, that the agency couldn't control the nation's AIDS research agenda.

A year after the research units were launched with such fanfare, Tony Fauci assembled an advisory committee to critique their progress. Its report called the development of the drug testing program "an assignment of enormous proportions," one "unprecedented in clinical research in this country." Thomas Merigan, a Stanford professor and advisory committee member, said NIAID had created "the most powerful clinical trials group for a single disease that this country has ever seen." But the committee had no illusions that everything was going smoothly and voiced some serious concerns.

In 1988, partly in response to the committee's recommendations, the system was restructured. Eventually, forty-seven testing sites, including fifteen pediatric units, were developed to form the AIDS Clinical Trial Group.

They ran big-money research at big-name academic centers. By comparison, their accomplishments were quite small.

WHAT'S WRONG WITH THE DRUG TESTING SYSTEM

Drugs to be tested had to be scored by several gatekeeping committees. After studying laboratory or clinical data on promising drugs submitted by researchers in industry, academia, or government, candidates were labeled by the ACTG executive committee as high, medium, or low priority, or as "not recommended for testing at this time." Occasionally a drug was also approved for evaluation only because it was already being widely used by people with AIDS.

All prospective drugs, including those tagged high priority, still had a long road to travel before reaching patients. The pentamidine story made that fact painfully apparent. Specialized committees, including ones that focused exclusively on antiviral therapies and treatments for opportunistic infections, AIDS-related cancers, and pediatric AIDS, which would supervise the actual trials, had their own ranking system. Once they decided which studies they wanted to conduct, however, the executive committee had to give its sanction before the exhaustive testing process could begin.

As with any clinical trial, a formal protocol also had to be written and the studies had to be approved by the FDA and a local institutional review board. A pharmaceutical manufacturer had to be found who would agree to produce enough drug to run a complete trial. Only after all these steps were completed—and assuming any number of other obstacles had been overcome—could patients actually be enrolled in the trial.

The ACTG system swayed back and forth between directed and investigator-initiated research. NIAID's original approach was to identify promising but unexplored scientific avenues, then contract with testing sites to execute the studies. That was a daring idea, one that flew in the face of traditional scientific thought. Most people in the biomedical research community believed the best discoveries emerged when scientists worked in an environment of unfettered creativity, not when they executed government mandates. They pointed to the remarkable advances of twentieth-century science as testament to the strength of investigator-initiated research. Summing up this sentiment in a *New Republic* article, Robert Bazell, a science correspondent for NBC, wrote: "The mention of directed research evokes a defensive cry from most biomedical scientists, who see it as an assault on their intellectual freedom. They say that politics, not science, will determine what is done in the laboratory."

And so the bureaucrats decided that researchers should be allowed to study whatever they wanted. That meant that the drugs most likely to make their way through the ACTG system were the ones that captured the imagination of a willing investigator. In fact, rules were written that actually barred government officials from telling investigators what trials to run. "The ACTG is a grant, not a contract," Fauci reminded his critics. "I can't legally say to them, 'You must do that.' I have to depend upon the initiative of the investigator."

Investigator-initiated research spawned its own troupe of critics. "The restructuring effort was designed to encourage investigator innovation, increase public disclosure, and leave no stone unturned in the fight against AIDS," wrote Barry Gingell of Gay Men's Health Crisis in remarks presented before a congressional hearing. "It is clear that NIAID has not accomplished this. Innovation appears to be continually discouraged. . . . There has been no increase in public disclosure, and decisions regarding drug selection and protocol development remains unilateral, with no input from the affected communities."

ACTG researchers also engaged in wasteful duplications of effort. Under the new system, professional jealousies flared, and scientists eager to make a name for themselves were known to cloak their findings in secrecy until they were ready to be published, instead of sharing data with their colleagues. The free rein given to investigators—to decide what they would research and where, when, and how they would publish the results—allowed such abuses to occur.

In May 1990, for example, a panel of sixteen scientists reviewed data from five studies and agreed that steroids prevented deteriorating lung function in people with AIDS and could reduce mortality by 50 percent. Six more months passed before the panel went public with that announcement. Only then did most physicians begin to use the lifesaving steroids in their AIDS practices.

Why did it take so long for the study results to be released? Partly, the delay stemmed from disagreements about how to phrase the findings and a reluctance to be too definitive. And, in fairness, the information was not suppressed completely; hints about the encouraging news filtered out in piecemeal fashion at various scientific conferences throughout the summer. But there was a more damning explanation for much of the delay, an explanation so enraging to Paul Meier, vice-chair of the expert panel, that he lifted the veil of secrecy that often shrouds scientific debate. Meier went to the press to reveal that a panel member, whom he refused to name, had deliberately stalled, that a man of science had declared shamelessly, "This must not come out until my paper is published."

At times, the study-what-you-wish approach also made the ACTG system appear to be functioning like a body without a head. Instead of being in the vanguard of biomedical research, NIAID sat passively on the sidelines waiting for investigators to approach with good ideas, and then to execute them at their own pace.

Larry Kramer contrasted that approach to the one he saw used in the movie business. He knew from firsthand experience that when Hollywood studios had a commercially viable idea, they didn't sit around waiting for someone to submit a script on it; someone was hired to write the script they wanted.

"We go to Fauci and say, 'Why aren't these things being studied?' " Kramer complained. "And he says, 'Because no one has submitted grants to study them.' We say, 'So what? You find somebody. Why don't you put somebody in charge?' "

Another major conflict between activists and researchers centered on the ACTG system's penchant for studying only antiviral therapies rather than drugs to treat opportunistic infections. Why would researchers put all their eggs in the antiviral basket when secondary infections were the actual killers? Why gamble on long-shot research instead of going for the better odds?

The scientific rationale for trying to disable the AIDS virus was that a drug that stopped the deterioration of the immune system would also prevent the onslaught of opportunistic infections. But the spectacular professional payoff that would accompany discovery of an antiviral was also an enticement. The researcher who could defeat the AIDS virus, or find a vaccine that prevented the dreaded infection altogether, was sure to bask in glory, most likely walking away with a Nobel Prize.

Personal ambition is a poor determinant of research priorities and it infuriated many. Antiviral research, said Martin Delaney, is "high tech, it is exciting, it is the leading envelope of research, but it has a very low chance of success." Meanwhile, opportunistic infections kept on killing people. Finding effective treatments for secondary infections would greatly enhance quality of life and might even keep some people alive long enough to try new antiviral drugs, should they eventually be developed. Yet powerful ACTG scientists initially awarded the Primary Infection Committee all the status and made the Opportunistic Infection Committee the stepchild of the system.

While the proper balance between antiviral and opportunistic infection research was being argued, the National Institutes of Health was coming under intense criticism for the close, lucrative, and often undisclosed ties many of its investigators had to pharmaceutical firms. Scientists seemed indifferent to the prospect that their own conflicts of interest could distort objectivity. While the issue went well beyond AIDS-related clinical trials, it hit home with many ACTG researchers.

Mark Harrington was astute enough to realize the problem was not gross corruption but something far more subtle and insidious. Harrington asked, "Sure, a scientist may think he is being objective, but what happens just knowing that a drug company is giving him thousands of dollars for his work or his staff or his lab?"

Mathilde Krim used even stronger terms to describe her reaction to scientists getting handouts from the very firms whose drugs they were testing: "Conflicts of interest are unethical and smell terrible. It's disgraceful."

Some believed Peptide T was a case in point. The drug had been invented in 1986 by a group of scientists at the National Institute of Mental Health (NIMH), led by Candace Pert, a highly respected brain researcher. Three separate Phase I studies showed the drug could inhibit HIV from attaching to CD4 receptors on the surface of human T cells and there were clear indications it also improved neurological function. Best of all, there appeared to be no toxicity.

Pert was convinced that the drug held tremendous promise; for the next five years, she dedicated herself to the task of getting it into trials. It was backbreaking work, as she learned when she appeared before an ACTG committee shortly after Peptide T's development. Instead of getting the enthusiastic response to her request for more research attention that she had expected, Pert says that her scientific reputation was torn to shreds. "They raked me over the coals," she recalls. "They screamed that it didn't work and insinuated that my results were a hoax."

Perhaps mere interinstitutional rivalry accounted for this attitude and for the unconscionable delay in scrutinizing Peptide T more closely; the drug was the passion of the National Institute of Mental Health, not the ACTG. Perhaps it was a matter of ego—the eminent virologists on key ACTG committees were certain they'd be the ones to find some magic bullet. But a more malevolent explanation may also have been involved: several ACTG investigators had financial interests in therapies that competed directly with Peptide T's mode of activity.

Not until March 1991 were pivotal Phase II studies of Peptide T launched. In the meantime eager patients turned once again to buyers' clubs for a drug they believed in. It was only because Pert eventually left her position at the NIMH to devote full-time energy to pursuing Peptide T that the research ever got off the ground.

Meanwhile, pressure to control conflicts of interest had begun to build. On Capitol Hill, elected officials threatened legislative action unless the National Institutes of Health imposed stricter standards on government-funded research, especially in university settings. Following a public meeting in June 1989, NIH drafted a set of long-sought-after guidelines that would have barred researchers from conducting NIH-sponsored clinical trials if they were consulting for an involved pharmaceutical company at the same time.

The NIH guidelines generated immediate and heated debate. Congressman Ted Weiss called them "strong minimum standards," but complained that big loopholes remained. "Many universities are blind to potential conflicts of interest among their own faculty and will probably rely heavily on exemption provisions," he said. The universities, predictably and by contrast, thought the proposals were inflexible and stifling and called the reporting requirements "onerous."

And members of the ACTG executive committee were indignant. In December, eight researchers signed a letter to Katherine Bick, the NIH official who had drafted the guidelines. They complained that her proposal could seriously threaten the entire government-sponsored research effort against AIDS, and underscored the three-pronged symbiotic interaction among government, academic scientists, and the drug companies.

"Nearly all the ACTG principal investigators have some industrial consultative arrangements," admitted the writers, claiming that "such consultations facilitate, rather than impede, proper conduct of ACTG trials."

Barring researchers from all financial ties to the drug companies could have dire consequences, they warned. "It is possible that the ACTG . . . would collapse because of investigator withdrawal and lack of pharmaceutical industry participation," warned the angry letter. "Disclosure, and not restriction, is the key to success. Eliminating consultation altogether is not the answer."

In the end, the protest from ACTG officials and other NIH researchers killed the conflict-of-interest guidelines. A few months after they were drafted, the whole proposal was shelved—and Katherine Bick, who was close to retirement anyway, left the agency under duress.

If it accomplished nothing else, however, the conflict-of-interest debate at least focused a spotlight on the close and often lucrative connections between researchers and drug companies. Fauci vigorously denied that AIDS research was in any way influenced by the financial holdings of the ACTG's executive committee, but admitted it might sometimes appear that way.

"Is it true we are doing mostly larger studies and fewer smaller ones?" he asked rhetorically. "Yes. Is it true that we are doing it because the people on the executive committee decide what studies they do because they have financial holdings in these companies? No. Do we understand how there could be that perception? Absolutely."

By the summer of 1990, Fauci had taken steps to change that impression by imposing disclosure requirements on all ACTG investigators. Under the new terms, financial ties to drug companies were still allowed, but they could no longer be hidden.

Pharmaceutical firms had their own reasons to be discontent with the government research effort. They had finally become convinced there was money to be made in AIDS. If for little else, the profiteers at Burroughs Wellcome deserve some credit for leading others down the streets of gold. By the end of 1991, sixty-four different companies were studying eighty-eight potential treatments, according to a survey by the Pharmaceutical Manufacturers Association. But they felt excluded from the planning and design of ACTG trials and distressed by the pace of data analysis. Therapies they submitted for initial evaluation kept disappearing. Sometimes the reason was logical: the drugs didn't hold much promise and had been given a low-priority score. Too often, though, they did have some potential, and yet they vanished into the bureaucratic maelstrom without a trace.

Gradually some companies began avoiding the centralized ACTG system, turning instead to community-based researchers or their own connections with academic investigators. In early 1990, ACTG researchers canceled a meeting of the drug-selection committee because not one company had submitted a single candidate for testing. In light of the desperate need and the numbers of chemical compounds that showed potential—just a few months earlier, ACT UP had identified ninety-nine such agents—the cancellation of the meeting was astonishing.

Mark Harrington got an inkling of just how discouraged the private sector was when he got a telephone call from a drug company official. Commenting about it in a later interview, Harrington wouldn't reveal the source of the call, but his story still sounded shocking. A firm had submitted a drug to the ACTG selection committee and was told it looked promising. But that good news was followed by some startling information. A spokesperson for the ACTG told the company it would have to do its own statistical analysis on trial results, plus supply the drug, provide nursing services to patients, and extend a variety of other costly support.

Uncertain about the remaining advantages of running its drug through the ACTG system, Harrington recalls that the official asked, "If we are providing all this, what are you providing?"

"We are giving you the cachet of an ACTG protocol number when the drug comes up for FDA review," admitted the investigator.

The company was infuriated by the arrogance of that response and pulled its drug from the ACTG system. Harrington didn't know whether the drug would ever get tested.

16

AIDS AND WOMEN, CHILDREN, AND MINORITIES

Compassion will begin in the small towns in the quiet country throughout America when people understand that people living with AIDS and HIV are just like us because they are us.

—BELINDA MASON, member,
National Commission on
AIDS, 1958–1991

ALONG WITH ITS OTHER FAILINGS, the ACTG system has never been able to enroll women, children, minorities, or drug users in AIDS clinical trials in anywhere near their proportion in the infected population. Because experimental trials have often provided the only source of treatment, exclusion from trials can thus hasten death. "Let me say that the epidemic is an affirmative-action killer," said Chris Sandoval, assistant director of San Francisco's Shanti Project, which provides support services to people with AIDS. "The disease does not recognize color, creed, national origin, sexual orientation, spiritual path, or political affiliation. It only knows that the host is a living and breathing human being."

In 1990, 77 percent of the participants in the government-sponsored trials were white, 10 percent were black, and 12 percent were Hispanic. While these figures were ever so slightly more equitable than a few years earlier, they still did not match the demographics of the epidemic. During the same year, just 52 percent of all newly diagnosed AIDS cases were white. Blacks made up 30 percent of the total, and Hispanics 17 percent.

True, trial design was not solely to blame. Researchers were also grappling with suspicions and hostility from minority populations. In the black communities of America, for example, clinical trials still evoked memories of the Tuskegee syphilis experiment. Hostility toward the motives of researchers still lingered. Mark Smith, a physician involved in AIDS research at the Johns Hopkins School of Medicine, learned more about that when he walked the Baltimore streets that surrounded the university and spoke with local residents. He discovered then that "many had learned as children that people from Johns Hopkins went out in the street at night to snatch black people off the street and put them in the basement to experiment on them."

Subtle extortion also came into play. Take the fact that clinical trials often provide primary health care to participants. From one perspective, that's an obvious perk. In poor and minority communities, where such services are sparse, the promise of decent medical care is a powerful incentive for enrolling. But is that fair? Compelling impoverished parents to enroll their child in an experimental drug trial to get access to good care, or advising a patient to sign up for a trial just to get free medications, obviously raises some disturbing ethical questions.

To illustrate the dilemma, Mark Smith described a former drug user with a blue-collar job and no health insurance. The man needed both AZT and aerosolized pentamidine, but could not afford them. Smith told him he qualified for a research study where his drugs would be paid for—and the man signed up at once. "Something in the back of my mind nags me about that encounter, because I am not sure that his consent was as free as we might like," Smith said.

As the demographics of AIDS began to shift, pressure grew to recruit a more representative population into trials. It didn't happen quickly.

❖   ❖   ❖

Most clinical research conducted in the twentieth century has been tainted by its embarrassing record of excluding women. Heart disease, the leading cause of death among women, is a classic example. Almost every major research study designed to prevent, diagnose, or treat heart disease during the past few decades has used exclusively male populations. One of the largest was the federally financed study, begun in 1982, in which 22,000 male doctors were monitored to determine whether taking an aspirin every other day prevented heart attacks. Six years later the results were announced: aspirin offered some protection against heart attacks.

Does it also prevent heart attacks for women? Since women get fewer heart attacks than men, the study would have had to enroll many more women, or taken even longer, to get conclusive results. Thus they were excluded, leaving researchers to guess whether the findings were equally applicable to women. It took four more years, and intense political pressure, before the NIH launched a study of 45,000 female nurses to answer the same question.

The history of AIDS research is no different. For both medical and socioeconomic reasons, the course that AIDS takes in women is markedly different from that in men, and women die more swiftly. Poor access to health care, few opportunities to participate in clinical trials, the absence of culturally appropriate educational information, and the burden of other caregiving responsibilities are all factors. There has not yet been a comprehensive study of all HIV-related illnesses and cancers in women, nor has there been a clear picture of the relationship between CD4 cell counts and characteristic female infections. Genital-tract and reproductive-organ infections are often associated with the virus, but are not included in official definitions of AIDS. And the research to determine what treatments work best for women just hasn't been done.

Moreover, because the CDC definition is a filter through which eligibility for AIDS-related government benefits must often pass, women are routinely disqualified from entitlement programs. A poster displayed on bus stops around New York City summarized the situation tersely: "Women don't get AIDS. They just die from it." It was not until 1993 that the agency formally redefined AIDS to include any HIV-infected person with a count of 200 or fewer CD4 cells.

While that adds thousands of women to the AIDS caseload, Social Security Administration number-crunchers promulgated new rules excluding many of them from receiving disability benefits—the opposite of the CDC's objective.

Sonia Singleton, age thirty, an HIV-positive Florida woman and a recovered drug addict, told her moving story to the National AIDS Commission in the spring of 1990. Three years earlier she had enrolled in a drug recovery program and had been tested for HIV—without her consent. Ever since, she had struggled to enroll in an appropriate clinical trial. But the ground rules kept shifting, and her qualifications never seemed to match those required by promising trials. "Read my lipstick," Singleton quipped before the commission. "Women do not have the same symptoms as men. Women have been systematically eliminated from research protocols testing new AIDS drugs. We still don't know how women are physiologically affected by AZT."

Singleton's articulate testimony highlighted a further inequity of the trial system. Excluding pregnant women from experimental trials, generally because of fears that a fetus would be damaged by poorly understood drugs, could be justified. But excluding all women of childbearing age because researchers didn't trust them to make rational decisions about getting pregnant was patently discriminatory.

"Either there are physiological and hormonal differences that are significant in the pharmacological effects of drugs on women versus men or there are not," said Nan Hunter of the ACLU. "If those differences do not exist, women should be afforded the right to participate in drug trials. If those differences do exist, then the drug should be tested in women. Otherwise, drugs would be eventually licensed for sale and use in the medical community without ever having been tested in women subjects first."

In a new twist, some later ACTG trials were specifically designed for pregnant women in hopes of preventing HIV transmission to the fetus. Sonia Singleton was confronted by a peculiar irony. "Two years ago I was unable to qualify because I was of childbearing age. Now it appears that I must be bearing a child to qualify for a research protocol," she said. Under the rules of one such trial, which used placebo controls to see whether AZT reduced the chance of transmitting the virus, women were dropped from the trial six weeks after they gave birth. At that point they lost their access to free medical care, and it became starkly clear that the research had never been designed with their needs foremost in mind.

Most often, the decision to exclude women from a trial was done simply to save drug companies money; if no women were enrolled, there were fewer liability concerns and there was no need to assess the risks of birth defects. Whatever the motive, the result was a further sense of desperation. Frantic to sign up for an experimental trial of Ampligen, an antiviral drug with the potential to bolster the immune system, one woman offered to waive any rights to a liability suit in the event of damage to a fetus. When that failed, she asked to be sterilized.

Under pressure from community health providers, infected women, and patient advocates, the first National Conference on Women and HIV Infection, sponsored by the Public Health Service, was held in December 1990. A few months later the ACTG established a Women's Health Committee to review appropriate research. Will it be enough? Taryn Lindhorst, who is involved with AIDS bereavement services in New Orleans, is not convinced.

Writing in the journal *Affilia*, Lindhorst described the social forces that diminish concern for women with AIDS: "In addition to sexism, which automatically devalues and obscures women's concerns at the societal level, is the 'courtesy stigma,' which silences discussions of women sufferers of a 'gay' disease. The American preoccupation with and devaluation of gay people and the gay culture, based on centuries of moral teachings that have reinforced homophobia, have ensured that most attempts to combat AIDS are bogged down in bigotry and reaction. When nongay people were diagnosed early in the epidemic, physicians routinely listed them as gay or bisexual, believing that AIDS could only strike this group. Thus, women with AIDS must contend immediately with the stigmatized nature of AIDS itself."

The parents and guardians of HIV-infected children also felt hopeless. Before cutting short their young lives, AIDS often ravages their brains. Their performance on IQ tests plummets. They forget what they had already learned. In one tragic story, a once-normal eight-year-old boy became almost autistic, losing his ability to speak or even cry.

Clinical trials of AZT showed the drug could reverse these early signs of dementia. But only a handful of children were ever enrolled in pediatric AZT trials, which began in 1987, a year after adult trials were launched. There was no Treatment IND established for pediatric use for 2½ more years. And it was May 1990 before the FDA finally said AZT could be labeled and sold for use in children. Until then, an HIV-positive mother with no symptoms of illness could obtain AZT, but her dying child could not.

Such happenstances were almost the norm in pediatric AIDS. As with the ban against testing drugs on prisoners, the reluctance to experiment on children or allow them access to unapproved medications had roots in a praiseworthy goal—protecting vulnerable populations who could not provide informed consent. But with AIDS, honorable intentions often lead to anguish.

One father who testified simply as "Joe" to maintain his privacy described his experience. After his sixteen-month-old daughter recovered from her first bout of *Pneumocystis carinii* pneumonia, she was put on pentamidine to prevent a recurrence. Then she developed hives and had to be taken off the drug. Soon afterward, Joe learned that trimetrexate was being tested against PCP. But his newly raised hopes were soon dashed when he discovered the trials were open only to adults. Joe was told that no other options existed for his daughter.

He was told one more thing: Just hope that the PCP does not come back. The implication was clear—nothing more could be done for her.

Then he heard about ACTG Protocol 045, the government's intravenous immunoglobulin (IVIG) study for children.

The immunoglobulin study was another example of the cruelty of rigid study designs. The trial was designed at the National Institute for Child Health and Human Development, a branch of the NIH, and was eventually subsumed within the ACTG structure. The nomenclature—Protocol 045—revealed nothing scurrilous. Its objective sounded benign: to determine whether intravenous immunoglobulin could safely and effectively prevent bacterial infections among HIV-infected children. Even the medical requirements did not sound outrageous: once a month the young participants would come to the hospital, where they would remain for four hours while a fluid slowly dripped through a needle into their arms.

But Protocol 045 was an outrage.

The study began in March 1988. Over the next 2½ years, 372 children, ranging in age from two months to twelve years, were enrolled at twenty-eight sites around the country. Half the children who came had a totally worthless fluid injected into their arms— hours of discomfort in their brief and tormented lives, with no prospect of gain.

There were several justifications for the placebo. Some scientists believed placebos were necessary both to demonstrate the drug's efficacy and to remove investigator bias. And, incredible though it sounds, some believed it was also necessary to expose two groups to the risk of contagious agents found in the hospital—one taking the drug and one not—in order to make direct comparisons between them.

Children testing immunoglobulin were also denied access to AZT. At the time, the drug was approved only for use in adults, but many pediatricians involved in Protocol 045 protested loudly that it should also be given to gravely ill children on a compassionate-use basis. It was not. No one on the trial got AZT until the FDA approved the Treatment IND for pediatric use in October 1989.

The immunoglobulin trial was closed down in January 1991, a year before its scheduled completion date. By then, researchers were confident that children getting immunoglobulin had fewer bacterial infections and were hospitalized less often than those who did not. It was an important finding, to be sure, but one that could almost certainly have been learned without using placebos.

If Protocol 045 did not violate the requirement, set down in the Nuremberg Code more than forty years earlier, that medical experiments avoid all "unnecessary physical and mental suffering and injury," it certainly came close.

Joe's daughter was growing weaker when he learned about Protocol 045. At first she didn't qualify for the trial because she didn't have the "right" infections; the study was designed to test the drug on HIV-infected children who had both a viral and a bacterial infection. By the time she did develop the appropriate infections, Joe would not allow her to participate because placebos were being used. "Who has time for placebos?" he asked, beseeching the researchers just to give his daughter the experimental drug. His pleas fell on deaf ears.

The child took a turn for the worse. No longer could she sit up on her own, take food, or speak. Her motor skills deteriorated to the level of a five-month-old, and her legs trembled. Desperate to do something to help the little girl, her physician called Burroughs Wellcome and asked to have AZT released to her on a compassionate-use basis. The company refused. Even Joe's offer to sign a waiver absolving them from a lawsuit failed to make a difference.

There wasn't much left to do. The PCP returned, and researchers finally said that if she survived the lung infection they would admit her into an experimental AZT study. By then it was too late. All Joe could do was plead for more humane ways to treat other children with AIDS in the future. "Let's not sit here and watch our children deteriorate before our eyes," he told congressional investigators. "I am watching my daughter do that right now, and I can tell you that it is a frustrating and horrible sight."

If the ACTG's record of minority participation in clinical trials was embarrassing, if the enrollment statistics for women and children were dismal, the contemptuous treatment afforded drug users was outright negligence.

In 1987, drug users represented some 15 percent of AIDS cases. At the time they were reasonably well represented in clinical trials; 12 percent of the enrollees were drug users.

Three years later the drug-using population accounted for a quarter of new AIDS cases. But, rather than increasing their representation in clinical trials, the numbers actually fell slightly, to just 11 percent of all participants.

Two explanations were offered for the reluctance to allow drug users to test new drugs—and thus for consigning them to what Nicholas Rango, head of the AIDS Institute in New York State, called "therapeutic nihilism." The first explanation was that they were shunned by the medical establishment and disdained by the public at large, making them perhaps the most marginalized members of American society.

A second explanation for the absence of drug users in trials was the knee-jerk assumption that they wouldn't comply with the requirements of clinical trials. That was a clear overstatement. The myth lingered that drug users always skip appointments and fail to take their medicine as instructed. The misconception has refused to fade despite studies that consistently discredit it. Actually, compliance is on a par with other population groups—especially when drug users are also enrolled in drug treatment programs.

Mostly it was social blinders that excluded drug users from experimental drug trials—the same social blinders that made it difficult for them to gain access to decent medical care, limited the availability of drug treatment, and stymied efforts to provide appropriate education and prevention. Together these blinders had to be blamed for an AIDS caseload among drug users that in 1990 rose faster than among gay men. Although there were still twice as many gay men as drug users diagnosed with AIDS—almost 28,000 gay men compared to about 10,000 drug users that year—by the end of 1990, the numbers of new cases among gays was up 19 percent from the previous year, while the caseload of drug users had grown by 24 percent.

Scientists had to do better. Excluding whole categories of sick people on the basis of color, sex, age, or behavior was "inappropriate social policy, bad public health practice, and poor science," said Wafaa El-Sadr, chief of infectious diseases at Harlem Hospital. While it was unfair to expect the ACTG system to solve all the far-reaching inequities of the American health care system—and, indeed, those of the society at large—it was proving impossible to ignore them. The proper balance between protecting vulnerable populations from abuse and denying them access to experimental drugs clearly had yet to be attained.

17

THE ILLICIT COMPOUND Q TRIALS

We may affirm absolutely that nothing great in the
world has been accomplished without passion.

—GEORG HEGEL,
Philosophy of History

The ruling passion conquers reason still.

—ALEXANDER POPE,
Moral Essays

THE ACTIVISTS WERE CONVINCED that the inability of the clinical trial
system to respond to their needs was constrained at least as much by
imagination as by science. Martin Delaney maintained that people
with AIDS and their advocates should not have to bargain with Mexican shopkeepers, fight with Japanese businessmen, or whip up unlikely concoctions in kitchen laboratories to get promising drugs. "We
don't pretend this is a good way to run an epidemic," said Delaney.
"I think we would all be better off if whatever treatments we had
were coming from legitimate, monitored pharmaceutical sources with
government approval."

The irony of those remarks became apparent in 1989, after a series
of underground trials were launched that carried patient autonomy to

a new level. In one of the most radical—and almost certainly illegal—moves of the epidemic, Martin Delaney and physicians in four American cities devastated by AIDS took it upon themselves to bypass many of the norms of medical research. They claimed they had been led to the point of desperation by the conviction that ACTG researchers could not swiftly test a promising drug.

By February 1989, the pipeline between Asia and the United States that had been laid during the heyday of the dextran sulfate boom was empty. As it became clear that patients could not absorb dextran sulfate properly, demand for the drug had trickled almost to a halt. The pipeline was soon to fill again.

Compound Q had been used in China for centuries to induce abortions and was also a component of many herbal remedies. An extract from a plant protein called trichosanthin, derived from the root of a Chinese cucumber, Compound Q first came to the attention of American scientists in 1987.

Hin-Wing Yeung, a biochemist from the Chinese University of Hong Kong, was visiting San Francisco back then. He told Michael McGrath, head of the AIDS immunology research laboratory at San Francisco General Hospital, about his work with trichosanthin. When McGrath heard that the drug had been able to target specialized immune cells, he became very excited and began trying to duplicate Hin-Wing Yeung's findings. Jeffrey Lifson, a scientist with GeneLabs, a biotechnology firm based in Redwood City, California, came onto the scene soon afterward and began working with McGrath.

Together the researchers developed a purified form of the drug, known as GLQ-223. Soon they were able to confirm that, in the test tube at least, trichosanthin could target and destroy HIV-infected cells while leaving healthy cells intact. The special appeal of Compound Q was that in addition to blocking replication of the virus in T-helper cells, it was effective against the reservoir of virus stored in macrophages.

Animal tests on Compound Q got under way. Almost two years passed before the researchers were granted an American patent on the drug, with Michael McGrath, Hin-Wing Yeung, and two GeneLabs scientists sharing inventorship credit. During the lengthy patent deliberations, the public was kept in the dark about a drug some experts hoped might actually be a cure for AIDS.

After preliminary results of the animal tests were published in the *Proceedings of the National Academy of Sciences,* the FDA gave its go-ahead to run Phase I clinical trials. Paul Volberding of San Francisco General Hospital was put in charge. Only a handful of patients, all in the advanced stages of AIDS, were enrolled in the study. Everyone was to get just a tiny dose of the drug. So far, everything was creeping along at the usual scientific pace.

The speed, however, was soon to pick up. Reports of the successful animal tests were leaked into San Francisco's gay community before they were published. Word spread quickly. Like ribavirin, isoprinosine, AL-721, and dextran sulfate, Compound Q was suddenly hailed as a likely cure, the next in a long line of alleged wonder drugs. A handful of patients soon managed to secure Compound Q through illicit sources.

Martin Delaney of Project Inform watched from the sidelines as excitement about Compound Q began to build. Then he called a meeting with Larry Waites, a pediatrician, and Al Levin, an allergist. Waites had closed his private office after losing a close friend to AIDS, and had soon teamed up to work with Levin, a political radical who had founded San Francisco's Positive Action Health Care, a private medical practice targeted at asymptomatic HIV-infected people.

Delaney, Waites, and Levin believed that Compound Q was far more promising than most of the drugs that had surfaced over the past few years, but also much more toxic. There were indications that the drug could cause mental confusion, seizures, coma, and death. Formal studies would take years to complete, and hundreds, perhaps thousands, of eager patients were likely to secure it through underground sources in the meantime. In explaining his leap into the fray of drug research, Delaney recalled, "Our fear was that if the drug was as helpful as we hoped, it would be forever before we got the answer on it. If it was as dangerous as we feared, large numbers of people could be hurt from self-experimentation."

Beneath the frustrations and concerns all three expressed at that meeting, one thought remained unspoken. Finally, someone said out loud what each of them had come silently to believe—they were going to run their own trial on Compound Q.

*   *   *

In the spring of 1989, the world watched on tenterhooks as tension mounted in Beijing's Tiananmen Square. AIDS activists arrived in Shanghai to court drug manufacturers just as government tanks rolled into the spiritual and political heart of China and cracked down viciously on the student activists.

Jim Corti—"Dextran Man"—again played the role of chief bootlegger. At Martin Delaney's request, Corti had tracked down the Shanghai factory where Compound Q was produced. But obtaining the drug took some doing.

After animal test results were published in the United States, the manufacturer had been besieged by requests for Compound Q and now claimed it was scarce. Corti suspected the claim was just a negotiating ploy. He knew that bribes were one of the costs of doing business in China. In response, he was silver-tongued, pressing his cause persistently until the manufacturer agreed to supply as much Compound Q as Corti wanted. The triumph was costly, but Corti had fortunately come well armed with cash. It took thousands of dollars to secure enough drug to put Martin Delaney's bold plan into action.

Meanwhile, back in the United States, Delaney, Waites, and Levin were ironing out the details of a four-city trial, under Project Inform's official sponsorship. They found physicians in New York, Los Angeles, San Francisco, and Fort Lauderdale who shared their conviction that desperately ill patients were entitled to take their chances on unproven drugs, so long as they were properly informed about them.

The underground trial of Compound Q officially began in May 1989. In New York, Barbara Starrett, who shared a private practice with her sister and saw mostly AIDS patients, persuaded a sympathetic minister at the Judson Church in Greenwich Village to hand over the keys to the basement every Tuesday night. Starrett arranged for beach chairs and had pizza delivered so that the mood in the church basement more closely resembled a community social event than a hospital ward. Patients who wanted to participate in the Q trial first had to sign an eleven-page consent form acknowledging the risks. Some consent statements were also videotaped.

Nonetheless, in launching its trial of Compound Q, Project Inform refused to play by traditional rules. The smuggled drugs had not met the FDA's rigorous standards for purity. Nor did the study have FDA sanction or the approval of local Institutional Review Boards (IRBs), which pass judgment on the ethics of a study. Despite its length, the consent form might not have withstood their scrutiny. Moreover, the underground researchers skipped the lowest doses in their Phase I trials, administering doses of Q that would not ordinarily have been used until Phase II.

On June 24, 1989, all of these irregularities took on new importance. Robert Parr, a former British fighter pilot, died that day in San Francisco.

In June, Parr became comatose two days after beginning treatment with Compound Q. Then he emerged from the coma and seemed to be recovering, but a few days later he aspirated his own vomit and died in his sleep. Suddenly the veil of secrecy that had covered the Project Inform study was stripped away. Although Parr's death was never directly linked to Compound Q, press attention across the nation nonetheless became riveted on the underground trial.

At first, Delaney claimed that Project Inform was just monitoring patients as they were treated, not conducting an official study. It seemed like a trivial distinction, but it was actually a shrewd legal maneuver. The FDA considers the "practice of medicine" almost untouchable; the agency regulates research, not what goes on in a doctor's office.

Delaney also reminded his critics that patient deaths were a common part of more traditional trials and asserted the FDA had been properly alerted to the underground testing of Q. Agency staff probed that allegation and claimed to find only one unofficial-looking and very vague document that described it, certainly nothing that met the FDA's detailed requirements for initial human trials. Delaney claims differently—he says a top FDA official actually had the detailed protocol. "When the story blew up in the press, this peron asked, 'Please keep my name out of this.' We did so to save this individual's highly placed, highly visible ass."

Delaney tried to make a case that the physicians involved in his study should be praised, not criticized, for acting to curb the indiscriminate use of a potentially toxic drug. Delaney's point was that a mainstream researcher like Paul Volberding, who was still conducting his own Compound Q study at San Francisco General, did not have the trust of the gay community. "He could talk until he was hoarse and the response is going to be, "Who are you to tell us what we can and can't do?" said Delaney, adding that the same message from a grassroots agency got a lot more respect. "When Project Inform said, 'Don't take this drug until we can learn more about it,' the gay community was more likely to listen."

The FDA didn't put quite the same spin on the Project Inform operation. Regulators thought Delaney had transcended the bounds of acceptable behavior. The agency launched an investigation into the Compound Q trial and the circumstances surrounding Parr's death.

The trials continued. Both Ellen Cooper and her boss, Carl Peck, director of the FDA's Center for Drug Evaluation and Research, believed they were illegal. But at the same time, more than ever they sympathized with patient frustrations and recognized that the issue could easily create political havoc, possibly weakening the uneasy truce that had settled in between the FDA and the patient activists by the summer of 1989.

Peck eventually wrote Delaney, asking that he stop the trials until formal FDA approval could be obtained. Peck's tone was conciliatory; he suggested Delaney come to Washington for a meeting at which the FDA would review Project Inform data. Then they could decide together about the next steps. That historic rendezvous took place in October 1989.

Once again the FDA was in a no-win situation. Had it chosen to come down hard on Project Inform, the agency would undoubtedly have been accused of being an overly rigid, heartless regulator. This time it took a more politically savvy approach and instead found itself under attack from mainstream researchers. Many were furious at the FDA's decision to have a collegial meeting with Project Inform rather than prosecuting the study organizers. "How dare the FDA imbue an unapproved trial with legitimacy by such a meeting?" asked one researcher, who said the FDA appeared to be sanctioning unauthorized studies.

Delaney himself had expected at least to have his wrist slapped at the Washington meeting and might well have deserved it, considering how far he had pushed the limits of the law. At the very least, he had jeopardized his credibility and might have been subject to legal action for his role in the underground Compound Q trial; perhaps he could even have been charged with a criminal offense in the death of Robert Parr.

No such thing happened. Ellen Cooper was said to be impressed by the early data, despite the absence of scientific controls. And Project Inform was advised to develop a protocol to continue and expand its trials—this time, taking traditional scientific principles more carefully into account. For Delaney, it was the best outcome imaginable, and he called it "a dream come true."

The Compound Q tragedies did not end with the death of Robert Parr. Two more patients died while on the first trial. One was a suicide, and no one linked it to the drug. Scott Sheaffer's death in New York was another story.

Sheaffer, a young actor, had first been given the drug in July. Three days afterward he became highly agitated, suffered temporary paralysis, and was hospitalized. Eventually he recovered and did not take Q again. Soon after, he became critically ill again and was back in the hospital by mid-August. By the end of the month, more than six weeks after his last dose of Q, he was dead.

Although Sheaffer had already had three bouts of PCP and numerous opportunistic infections, his lover was convinced that Compound Q had killed him, and took the story to the *New York Times*, which ran it on the front page. The death split the ranks of the patient activist community as few other events in the history of AIDS drug development had done. Critics said that Project Inform's underground trial was a desperate gamble—and the roll of the dice had come up craps. Michael Callen was especially critical because the study had not been given ethical sanction from an Institutional Review Board. Mark Harrington added that if activists were going to do their own research, they had to meet "the highest standards of scientific integrity and medical care."

But if Delaney was humbled, he was certainly not deterred, and he moved forward with plans for further trials. Over the next five months he spent a lot of time huddling with scientists trying to develop new designs.

On March 8, 1990, the FDA approved Project Inform's plans to continue testing Compound Q. At the same time, the agency broke the Shanghai connection by insisting that trials be conducted with

GLQ-223, the GeneLabs version of the drug. Sandoz Pharmaceuticals, which held worldwide marketing rights to the GeneLabs drug, gave Project Inform $250,000 to run the new study. In a compromise worked out with the FDA, the trial was open only to patients who had previously been treated with Compound Q. The idea was to give patients who already had faith in the drug continued access without opening the doors too much wider.

Unlike many other drugs, which had a scant fifteen minutes of fame before vanishing into the abyss of disappointing AIDS therapies, Compound Q continued to generate interest.

But Project Inform's scientific methods angered some mainstream researchers. Sparks flew during the San Francisco AIDS conference, when Delaney came head to head with Arnold Relman, then editor of the prestigious *New England Journal of Medicine.*

Delaney boasted about the early results of his Q study and defended the tactics that had kept it in the public eye for so long. "We've violated some sacred cows but have covered lots of ground in record time," he claimed.

Relman disagreed, and raked Delaney over the coals for making "premature" claims for the drug. He was also irate that Delaney had not submitted his data for peer review, and called Delaney's preliminary reports "black magic."

It was hard to judge who was right, because neither Project Inform nor San Francisco General Hospital, where Phase I trials were plodding along, was quick to publish its results. When preliminary studies from both groups were finally published in December 1990, in the same issue of the medical journal *AIDS,* the findings were tentative, as early studies usually are, agreeing conclusively only that additional research was necessary.

Still, in the time since the FDA shined a spotlight on Project Inform's first underground trial, the activists and the traditionalists had moved much closer together. Delaney admitted that he had been sobered by some of the realities of the scientific process, and he seemed more willing to listen to regulators and scientists. "Despite all the best intentions in the world and all the effort to cut corners, we saw it still takes so damn long to get answers out of clinical research," he said. "That was a profound learning experience."

The FDA, for its part, had approached the Martin Delaney/Compound Q problem with imagination, flexibility, and a determination not to be antagonistic. The agency's measured response had one especially remarkable result: it helped Martin Delaney take a step toward joining the system.

18

THE ddI MILESTONE

One does not discover new lands without consenting
to lose sight of the shore for a very long time.

—ANDRÉ GIDE

DESPITE THE FLAWED RESEARCH system that frustrated patients and
prompted the Compound Q experiment, the ddI trials progressed as
hoped. Parallel track and ddI were closely linked in the minds of the
public health community. Congressman Henry Waxman had observed that if parallel track worked, it could revolutionize drug development for some time. If it failed, it could cripple AIDS research.
Partly for that reason, the expanded distribution of ddI was closely
scrutinized by scientists, activists, and the drug companies. Everyone
knew that if the early drug distribution damaged enrollment in formal
ddI trials, or had toxic consequences, it would be hard to find anyone
willing to walk the same road a second time.

Two months after the innovative program was launched, Gina
Kolata, who covered the health beat for the *New York Times*, rang
alarm bells about it in an article that read: "Almost twenty times as
many people have flocked to free distributions of the new drug ddI
than have signed up for the clinical trial, leaving researchers in despair over whether they will ever be able to complete the formal
study."

At the time, only 75 patients had volunteered for the ACTG trials.
By contrast, 1,300 had already asked for the drug outside the trial.

Prominent researchers suddenly got the ammunition they needed to criticize the program. Douglas Richman, of the University of California at San Diego, called parallel track "an invitation to disaster." Jerome Groopman of New England Deaconess Hospital in Boston said, "If the philosophy is that anyone can decide at any point what drugs he or she wants to take, then you will not be able to do a clinical trial."

A few months later, more fuel was added to the fire of controversy. This time, Kolata wrote that patients taking ddI on the expanded-access program "have been dying at more than ten times the rate of those who are taking the drug in standard tests." The implication of the story was that patients were not being monitored as strictly as they would have been on a formal trial. The investigators who disliked expanded access immediately seized on the deaths as a reason to dismantle the whole program. Thomas Chalmers, a well-known public health expert from Harvard, was quoted as calling the high mortality rates in the program "a disgrace, an absolute disgrace."

Kolata immediately became the center of the story she had been sent to cover, and was nearly deafened by the roar of reaction to it. Its suggestion that the expanded-access program was a risk to safety led thousands of distraught patients to telephone their physicians in fear. According to David Barr, the Lambda attorney now with Gay Men's Health Crisis, enrollment in the formal trials fell sharply for the next two months as a direct result of Kolata's stories. Bristol-Myers's stock took a hit on the New York Stock Exchange. There was concern that the article would derail parallel track, and in one of four responses to it published in the *Times*, twenty-three AIDS community leaders signed a letter saying the front-page story would "jeopardize the lives of people with AIDS."

Kolata's piece became legendary in both scientific and activist circles, a classic example of how difficult it was to separate the politics of AIDS from the science. What she had largely overlooked was that many of the patients receiving ddI on an expanded-access basis were too sick to participate in clinical trials. Researchers sought participants likely to survive the length of the trial; most people getting the drug on the expanded-access program were running out of time.

Ultimately, expanded access to ddI neither proved to involve undue risks nor did it hamper enrollment in official trials. The ACTG system's early trouble in attracting patients turned out to be linked to its very strict eligibility criteria. One of the trials, for example, required people to have very low T-cell counts—below 200—yet to have been taking AZT for less than six months, a fairly unlikely combination. The pace of enrollment picked up considerably when those requirements were eased.

Meanwhile, distribution outside the trials had worked just as intended; it had gotten the drug into the bodies of patients with no therapeutic alternatives. Sam Broder was delighted with the speed at which ddI had been given out. "Because of urgency and pressure and compassion, things moved at a rate that was unbelievably fast," Broder said. "I think that's justified in people whose lives are at risk. If somebody is suffering or is in a life-threatening situation, you can afford to take certain chances."

Just what AIDS activists had been trying to tell the medical establishment for years.

On May 21, 1990, just one day short of three years since Treatment IND regulations had been published, the parallel-track policy proposal finally appeared in the *Federal Register*. It was structured to allow patients access to unapproved drugs only if they couldn't participate in a controlled clinical trial for one reason or another.

Although it was significant as evidence that the FDA had further loosened its grip on experimental therapies for life-threatening diseases, parallel track has not proved to be the final word on the issue of early access. For one thing, it is structured to be an option for the middle class and thus highlights the inequities of American health care, as AIDS so often does. In the Harlems of the nation, most poor people rely on public hospitals and community health centers for care, when they can get it at all. These institutions have repeatedly failed to distribute unapproved drugs because of the enormous amounts of paperwork involved and the potential liability risks. Furthermore, while therapies distributed through parallel track are expected to be free, other components of care essential to protect patients using experimental drugs—including primary care, lab tests, and ongoing monitoring—have prohibitive price tags for those with few economic resources.

Regulators at the FDA continue to believe that the push for parallel track was more a political maneuver by NIAID than a significant policy shift and mostly they still use Treatment IND to provide access to unproven therapies. But whatever Tony Fauci's initial motivation in proposing parallel track, the subsequent debate clearly helped prod the FDA into using the Treatment IND program more liberally where serious and life-threatening diseases are at issue. By December 1991, the agency had designated twenty-four Treatment INDs, including seven for AIDS-related drugs.

THE APPROVAL OF DDI

On October 27, 1990, in the waning hours of its fall session, the Senate approved the nomination of David A. Kessler, just thirty-nine years old, as Commissioner of the Food and Drug Administration. The post had sat vacant for more than a year after Frank Young's departure and the agency had been floundering without leadership.

Kessler had managed to secure his medical degree from Harvard Medical School, with a specialty in pediatrics, and his law degree from the University of Chicago almost simultaneously. He had run a hospital in the Bronx, where he had borne personal witness to the AIDS tragedy. And he had drafted legislation for Senator Orrin Hatch's Labor and Human Resources Committee, an experience that schooled him in the art of political compromises.

With his extraordinary intellect and his reputation for both compassion and pragmatism, Kessler seemed to bring a spirit of fresh hope to an agency demoralized by scandal and resource shortfalls. At least during his first year, Kessler had a honeymoon period with the press and with Congress. Everyone seemed eager to support the new commissioner, whose first order of business was to bolster respect for the FDA.

The activists were already lobbying for the licensing of ddI before Kessler came on board. Despite the drug's widespread availability, activists wanted the official stamp of FDA approval even before Phase II trials were complete.

Martin Delaney wrote a long letter to Ellen Cooper and her colleague Paul Beninger explaining why he believed that the drug—as well as ddC, a sister antiviral medication being developed by Hoffman–La Roche—should be approved. A letter signed by more than

150 patient advocacy groups made essentially the same demand. And shortly after his swearing-in, Kessler was also handed a citizen's petition demanding the licensing of ddI and ddC.

The activists thought the FDA was waiting for proof that both ddI and ddC were at least as effective as AZT. Since thousands of people were intolerant of AZT and had no other pharmaceutical options, they wanted a different standard to be used. "The proper hurdle," wrote Delaney, "should instead be reasonable proof of some degree of efficacy, however limited, against HIV. . . . I believe the case can and should be made that both ddI and ddC have already cleared it."

In the end, Delaney got his wish. But it took the aggressive efforts of FDA regulators to grant it.

What Delaney had perhaps not realized was that Bristol-Myers had approached the FDA in November 1990 with the news that it intended to submit an application for drug approval based solely on Phase I trials. That was extraordinarily unconventional since those early trials were intended mostly to assess the drug's safety, not its effectiveness, and lacked proper controls.

In strong language, the FDA advised Bristol-Myers to find a historical control, a population group that had never taken ddI but had characteristics similar to those that had, so that appropriate comparisons could be made. The company was warned that if it did not produce such a control, the FDA might well refuse even to file the application, instead bouncing it right back into the company's lap.

At the same time, pressured by a combination of genuine compassion and political concerns, the agency began looking for information that could corroborate the Bristol-Myers Phase I study and allow ddI to be approved. Much of the justification for the unprecedented actions that followed came from the Sub-Part E regulations promulgated in the fall of 1988, which had codified procedures for evaluating the safety and efficacy of certain drugs—and which initially and unfairly had been dismissed by activists as so much bureaucratic harrumphing. Those regulations state that in the case of drugs for serious and life-threatening diseases the "FDA has determined that it is appropriate to exercise the broadest flexibility in applying the statutory standard"; ddI clearly represented an occasion to exercise that flexibility.

Long before Bristol-Myers's application for approval was complete, FDA scientists asked the company for an early look at its raw data so that they could begin their own analyses. DdI Phase I findings were also summoned from Robert Yarchoan and Philip Pizzo, researchers at the National Cancer Institute. So urgent was the push to approve ddI that the agency also broke into ACTG Protocol 117, a Phase II trial in which AZT was being compared to ddI and which was at least a year from completion.

Securing permission to scrutinize an ongoing trial was a colossal effort that involved winning over some very uneasy people on the ACTG's executive committee. Carl Peck, director of the Center for Drug Evaluation and Research, who temporarily assumed leadership of the agency's antiviral division after Ellen Cooper's departure in December 1990, underscored just how remarkable it was to interrupt an ongoing trial. "It is usually FDA that is cautioning about the statistical hazards of premature or interim analysis," he said. "Nevertheless, exceptional acts may be warranted in exceptional circumstances. . . . Let me emphasize that we view the present peek at ongoing clinical trial data to be an extreme exception, certainly not to become the rule."

In perhaps the most important precedent set by the ddI review, the FDA accepted surrogate markers as an instrument for measuring the drug's effectiveness. Traditionally, the value of drugs for life-threatening diseases is measured by how long they allow a patient to survive. But death is a brutal endpoint; it forces researchers to wait years before they are sure whether patients using an experimental drug have died more slowly than those taking the control. By contrast, surrogate markers allow scientists to count improved health, signs of an enhanced immune system, or reduced viral activity as evidence that a drug works.

In the case of ddI, the FDA focused mostly on whether the drug improved CD4 cell counts. The decision to adopt that surrogate was not made lightly because its value in predicting patient health was uncertain. Under Peck's guidance, the FDA consulted widely with experts on the subject and eventually pioneered novel techniques for assessing ddI's impact on CD4 counts.

Thus the groundwork was already in place to consider the ddI application when it was submitted to the FDA on April 2, 1991. Four medical reviewers were assigned the full-time task of reviewing the data, whereas typically just one scientist would get the job. Their mandate was to move swiftly; an FDA advisory committee scheduled for mid-July would decide whether to recommend approval. By the time the players assembled for that meeting, held in Bethesda, where the merits of parallel track had been debated less than two years before, nearly 2,400 patients were enrolled in clinical trials in the United States and more than 4,500 were participating overseas. Almost 23,000 other people were getting free ddI through the expanded-access program.

David Kessler opened up the advisory committee hearings with words of praise for his own agency and then he set out the FDA's ambitious agenda for the future. "Our goal is to turn protocols around in weeks and to measure review times in months," he said. Kessler also thanked others who had helped move the review process forward swiftly, specifically mentioning Bristol-Myers, NIAID officials Tony Fauci and Dan Hoth, who had orchestrated the FDA's sneak preview of Protocol 117, and the activists.

"What we have been seeing is unprecedented cooperation," commented Kessler. "Let me also say that we have learned much from the AIDS community. We have recognized that FDA is, that we must be, accountable for what we do. . . . I think also that in some ways the AIDS community has gained a more complete understanding of the challenges that the FDA must confront. I appreciate the frank and open dialogue we have had with the AIDS community during the last several months. I would like it to continue."

On that note of optimism the presentations began. The first day was dominated by Bristol-Myers, which described its Phase I trials in detail. The data's weaknesses were painfully apparent. Had there been nothing else to consider, the committee would almost surely have had to turn down the drug—the rigorous requirements to prove safety and efficacy had clearly not been met. Toward the end of the eleven-hour session, Theodore Eickhoof, an advisory committee member from the University of Colorado in Denver, asked a question that went to the heart of the dilemma. "It is difficult to identify any strengths in the characteristics of the data base except speed and rapid turnaround, which is obviously one of the goals. Are we willing to pay the price in uncertainty?"

The following morning FDA scientists stepped forward to present their findings from months of legwork and managed to salvage the application. The early look at Protocol 117 and the FDA's use of surrogate markers proved invaluable. Agency reviewers had also tried to confirm the drug's safety by looking at data collected from patients getting ddI through the expanded-access program, but were somewhat disappointed. Because the program had not been designed with data collection in mind, there was too much inconsistency in the findings to be of great value. Still, an agency that had once been criticized for interpreting the Treatment IND regulations too narrowly now went on record as being willing to weigh data from expanded-access programs in the future, so long as it was properly collected.

The FDA's presentation helped bolster the confidence of the advisory committee. An extra measure of persuasion came from Donald Abrams, the community-based research pioneer who was also a member of the committee. Abrams put the issue in its proper context. "I think it is wise to point out that we are in the midst of a medical emergency. One person dies of AIDS every eight minutes in the United States today. . . . Many of these people are back in 1985 when there was nothing available to them."

In the end, the committee gave its blessing to ddI by a vote of 5–2, with one abstention. The stage was set for full FDA approval, which came for both adult and pediatric use on October 9, 1991, with the proviso that when the ACTG's Phase II results became available in the spring of 1992, the drug would be pulled from the market if its effectiveness was not confirmed. Bristol-Myers announced at once that the drug would be priced at $1,745 per patient per year, less than one-fifth the original price of AZT.

Kessler, who had earlier called on the ddI advisory committee to be creative, said the decision highlighted the FDA's new proactive stance. The development and innovative approval of ddI, claimed the commissioner, was a "milestone of drug review" and "the paradigm of the future." The FDA finally was shaking itself free from the sort of uncompromising approach it had demonstrated with ganciclovir. Many years before, Mathilde Krim had said "the FDA had to learn to distinguish between drugs for headaches and drugs for a deadly disease." Now, it seemed to be doing just that.

o   o   o

The insistence that Bristol-Myers halt sales of ddI if the ACTG results did not confirm the drug's promise was yet another atypical move in a highly unusual process. But it was a big improvement from the most likely alternative—turning down ddI altogether. Almost everyone agreed the drug's value had not been proved with certainty. "In my opinion, the data do not demonstrate that ddI is clearly clinically effective in treating adults with HIV infection," Clifford Lane, a NIAID researcher, told the committee. "I think there is a reasonable chance that it is effective. Given the need to have alternative therapies, I would strongly support allowing this drug to be marketed, but if there ever was a situation where you would have conditional approval, this is the place to put it in."

From that novel limitation emerged a new initiative to make experimental drugs more readily available to desperate patients. In November 1991, the FDA announced a proposal for "accelerated approval" of promising pharmaceuticals for serious and life-threatening diseases. The concept was that, like ddI, drugs would be approved for sale—and thus would presumably be covered by insurance companies—while testing continued. Under the proposal, which goes much further than existing expanded-access mechanisms, any therapy that failed to live up to its early promise would be swiftly removed from the market.

If it is implemented, accelerated approval will be yet another regulatory milestone for the FDA.

19

CRASHING THE GATES
Activists Enter the Drug Testing Sanctum

> Medicine, professedly founded on observations, is as
> sensitive to outside influence, political, religious,
> philosophical, imaginative, as is the barometer to the
> atmospheric density.
>
> —OLIVER WENDELL HOLMES

ALTHOUGH THE DDI STORY highlighted the remarkable shifts at the
FDA, the ACTG system still had to be prodded into greater responsiveness. Mainstream researchers were put off by the excesses of the
activists and had not yet been persuaded that patients should have a
voice in designing and executing clinical trials. They were not going
to change unless they were forced to do so.

But eventually they discovered that patients held a crucial bargain-
ing chip—their bodies. The researchers could not run trials without
their participation. Knowing they held that singular advantage, patients educated themselves in the arcane details of scientific studies
until they were prepared to negotiate with investigators on equal
footing. Much tactical maneuvering and many bitter words had to

come before some of the investigators were willing to accept patient advocates as their peers.

Mark Harrington spearheaded the effort to win Fauci's permission to attend ACTG meetings.

At a meeting in March 1989, the same one that had prompted him to begin complaining publicly about Treatment IND, Fauci told Harrington that ACT UP could participate in the ACTG meetings. His thinking at the time was that giving the organization a voice in designing clinical trials—and effectively bringing it inside the system— might help make research more attractive to AIDS patients. ACT UP had the foresight to videotape his agreement, a precaution in case those in the government bureaucracy should decide to reconsider their promise.

Many months passed before Fauci's pledge was actually implemented. In the interim there were a lot of hard feelings.

Tony Fauci has a habit of making rather loose promises. And why not? He wasn't going to have to explain his decision to the big-name ACTG scientists, a rather conservative group accustomed to traditional ways. That task, instead, was left to his underlings, mostly to Dan Hoth, the NIAID official who oversaw the clinical trial system.

Hoth wanted badly to earn the respect of the ACTG investigators. Pressuring them to open their forum to a group of boisterous radicals wasn't an effective entree, and Hoth balked at the whole idea. He tried to discourage ACT UP, and explained how uncomfortable scientists become when lay people attend their meetings. To deflect activist pressure, Hoth emphasized that he was just asking for a little more time to push open the doors. He asked ACT UP to skip the session scheduled for July 1989, but promised representatives they could attend the one that followed. ACT UP was amenable.

Four months later, in October, hundreds of ACTG investigators, pharmaceutical company officials, and other major AIDS research players were scheduled to meet again. The issue of activist involvement in the drug research system began to heat up. The week before the Bethesda conference, Mark Harrington telephoned Peggy Hamburg, Fauci's special assistant, and asked, "Where is our invitation?"

"I'll look into it," he was told. A flurry of telephone calls followed. Faxes were fired back and forth. Finally, ACT UP learned the ACTG investigators were still unwilling to have them attend. Fauci and Hoth hadn't made any meaningful progress in bringing the ACTG investigators on board and apparently hoped the issue of community attendance at scientific meetings would just fade away. They hadn't learned the full extent of ACT UP's tenacity.

With characteristic chutzpa, Harrington gave Fauci a lecture-by-fax about upholding his end of their bargain. His sign-off statement was not a threat, but a promise—even without official sanction, ACT UP would make its presence known, he wrote.

A few days later, five determined ACT UP representatives—Mark Harrington, Jim Eigo, Ken Fornataro, Iris Long, and Rebecca Smith—arrived at the Bethesda hotel where the investigators were meeting. Dan Hoth had begun his introductory speech by the time they walked into the conference room. He began by boasting about the accomplishments of ACTG's two major AZT trials, Protocols 016 and 019. Knowing the ACT UP interlopers had arrived, Hoth then turned his wrath toward them, laying down some ground rules in the process. As Harrington remembered it, Hoth said, "The issue of community participation has been precipitated by ACT UP New York. We didn't invite them and we wish they weren't here, but they are here and we have decided to try to avoid the danger of a physical confrontation by allowing them to attend all open meetings. However, they will not ask questions nor be allowed to talk."

It was a tense and discouraging three days. Harrington was angered by the attempts to muzzle him. Everyone resented the sudden decision to label some meetings "private," an obvious attempt to keep ACT UP in the dark. Another blow was the announcement that responsibility for collecting data for the ACTG trials was being transferred from the Research Triangle Institute in North Carolina to a group affiliated with the Harvard School of Public Health—and that in the interim, no major new trials would get under way.

"The cumulative picture that emerged was hostility, double-dealing by NIAID, control by a small number of principal investigators in a few select committees, immense frustration from scientists in other committees, suspicion and downright opposition to parallel track," said Harrington. "And finally, hearing that things had been screwed up so badly that the whole data operation would slow the system down for six to nine months gave us the idea that the ACTG was dead in the water."

Harrington was infuriated by the experience, and when he got home, he lashed out in his regular column in *Outweek*, the now defunct weekly magazine for New York's gay community. He titled the piece "In the Belly of the Beast" and compared the German debate over the opening of the Berlin Wall to the tempest stirred up by efforts to open up ACTG meetings. The Germans, wrote Harrington, had shown a good deal more grace.

Tony Fauci called Harrington after his *Outweek* piece appeared and asked him to tone down the rhetoric. "You don't know how hard we are trying to get you in," said Fauci.

Eventually, mostly in response to continued pressure, the ACTG leadership came around to the idea of community representation. Initially the activists had to content themselves with a single advisory committee, to be called the Community Constituency Working Group. The working group met for the first time in December 1989 with twelve community leaders from around the country. Soon after, in response to further prodding, the group was doubled in size, with increased representation from minority groups and more HIV-infected people.

ACT UP felt the working group represented little more than tokenism. Harrington was especially miffed that Core Committee and Executive Committee meetings, where most of the key decisions were made, still took place behind closed doors. Ever the rabble-rouser, he wanted more visibility; specifically, Harrington was pushing for two consumer representatives on every ACTG committee and three on the executive committee, each with the same decision-making authority accorded the scientists. Without their presence, the activist's were convinced the "Gang of Six"—Douglas Richman, Thomas Merigan, Martin Hirsch, Margaret Fischl, Paul Volberding, and Lawrence Corey—would remain in charge. As members of ACTG's Primary Infection Committee, they were the ones in search of the golden ring: the antiviral drug to conquer HIV.

Despite their warm relationship with Tony Fauci, activists kept attacking his research apparatus.

Larry Kramer's comments were blunt. "The ACTG system is

money down the toilet," he said. "It has already pissed away a billion dollars [actually, the figure was less than half of that at the end of 1991] and they've come up with essentially nothing."

Kramer's position, if extreme, reflected a widespread perception that the ACTG research record was dismal. ACT UP began hollering about its failures at any available public forum. ACT UP and other patient advocates claimed old drugs were being tested inefficiently and new drugs not at all.

Eventually, an ad-hoc coalition of twenty-five AIDS groups and other health organizations, representing a wide spectrum of political opinion, was formed. In early 1990 the group—which included many who had lobbied in favor of parallel track and against the high price of AZT the summer before—decided to fight for changes in how the government conducted its AIDS research. They demanded better coordinated and more adequately funded research, and called again for the inclusion of more women, children, drug users, and minority people in clinical trials, as well as greater study design flexibility and a focus on drugs for opportunistic infections.

While their lobbying efforts were under way, ACT UP continued to be an unwelcome presence at ACTG meetings. On several occasions, security guards forcibly ejected demonstrators from closed committee sessions. Also at this time, Mark Harrington was working hard to finish a critique of the ACTG system. With assistance from Jim Eigo, a preliminary draft of a heavily footnoted, sixty-seven-page document was ready in time for the March 1990 ACTG meeting. In that paper, ACT UP came down hard on the whole research apparatus. Some 200 copies of the draft were passed out to investigators attending the scientific session, with requests for comments. But its tone was hostile and there were few responses. Jack Killen, who worked closely with Dan Hoth, was reportedly angered by the document's innuendos and complained to Harrington about uncalled-for "character assassinations." Then Killen suggested Harrington resign from ACTG's patient constituency working group.

Although Killen eventually softened his words by suggesting that Harrington would be more effective as an outsider, the hard-to-subdue activist decided to fight for his seat. Harrington quickly arranged a conference call with other members of the working group and got their pledges of support. Matters heated up further when Jim Eigo threatened to resign from an Institute of Medicine panel. Eigo's threat was not directly linked to Harrington's tenure on the working group, but the timing of Eigo's announcement apparently disturbed Fauci anyway, who thought Eigo was "sensational."

Quite soon, Fauci got his chance to ask Harrington to stay. The occasion was another dinner at the home of Jim Hill, NIAID's deputy director. The circumstances that surrounded it were a bit odd. Peter Staley and Mark Harrington had called Fauci a few days earlier, told him they planned to be on the NIH campus and suggested an informal get-together. Fauci made the social arrangements, and when they arrived for dinner that evening, he greeted them warmly.

"What brings you down here?" he asked.

Harrington answered candidly. "We're taking pictures of the NIH campus for a demonstration in May."

Fauci learned that moment that he was to be the target of another noisy ACT UP demonstration. He realized—and not for the first time—that the personal rapport he had worked so hard to cultivate with the patient advocate community would not spare him from a public roasting. The activists still intended to hold him accountable for the clinical trial program.

If the men thought Fauci would lose his cool, they were disappointed. As usual, he kept a tight rein on his emotions. Fauci leaned back in his chair and calmly asked his guests if they really believed such an approach was likely to be effective. Whatever he thought of their answer, he decided not to press the issue, or to try to dissuade them from staging their demonstration.

In fact, the conversation soon shifted to other topics and lightened up considerably. As Harrington recalled the evening, "It was one of those funny encounters that you get in AIDS where you are supposed to be with your adversary but you are actually enjoying yourself."

During dinner, Fauci promised Harrington he'd have a chat with Jack Killen. A few days later, the telephone rang at Harrington's home. Jack Killen was on the line, calling to report a change of heart. Harrington was welcome to remain on the patient constituency working group, Killen said.

Shortly after the dinner ended, Jim Hill also got his chance to behave like a gentleman. At Hill's house that night, Mark Harrington accidentally left his notebook with all the plans for the demonstration.

In espionage circles, that was akin to a Soviet secret agent leaving his list of contacts at a White House dinner. But these men were playing by the rules of a more lenient game. Hill returned Harrington's notebook the next day.

ACT UP's critique was polished and in final form in time for the May 1990 ACTG meeting. This time, when ACT UP representatives wandered through the hallways passing out the fat report, ACTG researchers knew what was coming. Harrington tried to hand it to Dan Hoth, who stuck his hands into his pockets and refused to take it.

By then, it didn't matter much. Plenty of other ACTG members had been given copies of the revised document, and so had the press.

ACT UP's criticism generated enough negative publicity to provoke a response. In a paper called "NIAID Responds to ACT UP Allegations and Demands," the institute discussed its accomplishments in detail, prominently highlighting the completed AZT trials. NIAID defended its record on opportunistic infections and cancer therapy research, explained how doctors were notified about drug trial results before they were published, and highlighted constituent input into the ACTG process. The agency also put a familiar spin on the conflict-of-interest issue, crediting the success of many decades of biomedical research to the long-standing collaboration among government, academia, and industry.

Charges and countercharges were flying in late May, just before ACT UP's long-planned demonstration.

The action at the National Institutes of Health came on May 21, 1990, a year and a half after ACT UP had staged its noisy protest at FDA headquarters in Rockville, Maryland, virtually shutting down operations for the day.

Taking aim at NIH involved more than just a change of subway stops. It also reflected a determination to become involved in the drug development process at a much earlier stage. From a public-relations perspective, that decision had always been risky; NIH-related issues revolved around scientific judgment and they were complex, especially to a public with a short attention span. As John James wrote in *AIDS Treatment News*, "It is harder to organize people around

deaths caused by drugs which do not exist and perhaps never will, but
should."

Perhaps for that reason, just 1,000 people turned out for the demonstration, one-third the number its leadership had hoped for. Larry
Kramer was bitterly disappointed. "Very few people arc still doing
most of the fighting," he said. "For all of ACT UP's growth, we've still
got very small forces to call on. Everyone seems to be tired—or
dead."

Still, the protest was dramatic—interesting theater, Fauci said. A
chanting crowd marched onto the tranquil NIH campus, blocking
traffic along the way as they yelled, "Ten years, one billion dollars,
one drug, big deal," and "Storm the NIH." Some carried cardboard
tombstones, others placards that read "We Will Not Rest in Peace,"
and "One AIDS Death Every 12 Minutes." Bombs spewing purple
and green smoke were released on the grounds. Before it was over,
four hours later, eighty-two people had been arrested, beginning with
Peter Staley, who leaped onto the roof of a building and had to be
forcibly removed. Twenty-one other ACT UP protestors trooped
down the road to Rockville, where they occupied Dan Hoth's office
until they were escorted out in handcuffs.

Coincidentally, the Public Health Service's proposed parallel-track
policy was published in the *Federal Register* the day after the demonstration. The announcement came a full year after Fauci had first
proposed this new system of expanded access. But if the year-long
delay had been excessive—and had generated a barrage of criticism—the timing of the announcement was a stroke of good fortune
for AIDS activists. By linking the two stories, the press helped to bring
greater public attention to the whole issue of access to AIDS drugs.

Three days later, Fauci was on his way to New York to face some
of his sharpest critics.

A SEAT AT THE TABLE

Fauci had been scheduled to speak at the Fashion Institute of Technology long before the demonstration took place. His talk was supposed to be about treatment options for people infected with HIV but
exhibiting no symptoms. The audience, though, was packed with

ACT UP members and, predictably, more controversial issues were soon raised.

"I enjoyed so much the visit of some of you a few days ago," Fauci quipped. After describing NIAID's research priorities for the upcoming year, he fielded questions from a panel of experts, which included Kevin Armington of Gay Men's Health Crisis, ACT UP's Jim Eigo and Iris Long, Derek Hodel of the PWA Health Group, and a host of others. Again and again—especially when he was asked why so few trials were open to asymptomatic HIV-positive people and why ACTG studies emphasized antiviral medications—Fauci reminded the panel of the agency's limited resources and the need to set priorities.

He also tried to convey the awkwardness of deciding when to release information about promising drugs to the public and complained about being "damned if you do and damned if you don't. If you let the information out before it gets published, you are accused of popularizing. If you don't let it out, you are accused of undue delay."

Iris Long pushed Fauci on the underrepresentation of women and minorities in ACTG trials, reminding him that "the demographics of the disease and the demographics of the ACTG do not match." Fauci admitted the need to do better and pledged that changes were being planned. To that promise, Eigo responded dryly, "I continue to hope, but history tells me I'm a fool for doing so."

Then Fauci fielded questions from the crowd. The mood was far from friendly, and some of the threats were thinly veiled. "The drugs you've tested haven't worked," shouted one man. "Why don't you try the ones we've been begging you for years?" He was thinking at the time of a list developed by ACT UP, which included sixty antiviral drugs and dozens of therapies to boost the immune system, treat HIV-related cancer, and attack opportunistic viruses, fungi, and protozoa.

In pleading for a bolder response to the AIDS epidemic, another man warned, "If you can't find the profile in courage that I've seen all around me, in my own community, then I'm scared of what we may have to be driven to do to make you wake up. I hope it doesn't come to that."

The most moving moment of the evening came when one man

stepped to the microphone and asked, "If you had heard promises year in and year out . . . if you are still carrying the best friends you've ever had from churches or synagogues in caskets . . . if you're scared to death of getting sick yourself . . . what would you do, Dr. Fauci? What would you do?"

Fauci could not match the emotional tenor of the man's question, and his response was subdued. "I'd be very upset," he said. After the lecture, Fauci huddled with Peter Staley, Jim Eigo, Mark Harrington, and others, and invited them back to Bethesda.

The meeting took place several weeks later. ACT UP had pledged to be a noisy presence at the international AIDS conference scheduled in San Francisco for the end of June 1990, and Fauci wanted to meet with leaders of the group first. His goal was twofold: to have activist concerns addressed directly by his program staff and to expose his staff to the intense and building anger within the affected communities.

For five hours, Dan Hoth, Jack Killen, Maureen Myers, and other top NIAID representatives faced off against Harrington, Eigo, and David Barr.

The activists kept saying the ACTG was not testing enough drugs. Fauci told them they did not really understand the strengths of the ACTG system, and charged them with being unrealistic about available resources. Reflecting on that meeting later, Fauci said, "They went a little too far because they said the whole system stinks. We said the system as it's built is meant to answer broad questions. We are not going to tear that down."

Ever the master of compromise, Fauci also proclaimed his willingness to seek common ground, telling the activists, "You are absolutely correct, we should be doing a couple of other things." Then he repeated a past promise to create a mechanism that would allow one or two ACTG sites to conduct rapid-fire, small-scale tests on promising agents.

Fauci also underscored his intention to integrate the activists further into the ACTG process, including giving them a voice on the executive committee. "My goal is to have a very solid representation, not figurehead window dressing," he said.

In exchange, Fauci wanted the rhetoric toned down. "If they are trying to get into the system, they may have to modify some of their activist modes, but that doesn't mean that they have to become Uncle Toms." What he really wanted was a little support for NIAID's role as mediator. He was tired of the struggle to bring the sometimes rigid ACTG investigators and often flamboyant activists to the negotiating table—especially right after the activists had charged the researchers with murder or burned them in effigy.

Fauci kept his word. By November 1990, NIAID announced that every ACTG committee and working group would include patients and community constituents. The Executive Committee was enlarged from ten to twelve members to accommodate the broadened representation. Each one of the core committees, including the influential Primary Infection Committee, was also augmented.

But the much-longed-for therapeutic breakthrough failed to materialize. Larry Kramer was more convinced than ever that the problem with the ACTG system remained entrenched bureaucracy. "All the checks and balances in the system seem to cancel each other out," he said. "It took us years to get in the front door and it has been a most revealing and tragic peekaboo inside. There are so many knots in the system it can't respond."

Mathilde Krim, hardly an apologist for NIAID, disagreed. Her long-standing commitment to AIDS research gave her an insider's viewpoint on developments within the clinical trial system. "I can see incremental progress. We're making changes," she said, acknowledging that a cure or an effective vaccine remained a distant hope. Then she gave a revealing explanation for the difference between her quiet optimism and Kramer's bleakness, for her willingness to be patient and his desperate sense of urgency. "The difference is I'm healthy and Larry Kramer is sick."

CONCLUSION

❖

When I look back upon the past, I can only dispel the
sadness which falls upon me by gazing into that happy
future when the infection will be banished. . . . The
conviction that such a time must inevitably sooner or
later arrive will cheer my dying hour.

—IGNAZ SEMMELWEIS,
Etiology

IT HAS BEEN MORE THAN A DECADE since AIDS first darkened the
American landscape, but the reality of a quick medical fix remains
remote. Even if the federal government hands researchers a blank
check, a cure will likely remain elusive.

Part of the reason is that scientific progress takes time. But have the
limits of knowledge been reached? Has the development of new
therapies matched the pace of expanding scientific information?

In the early 1980s, the answer was an emphatic no. The absence of
aggressive leadership from the White House and the Department of
Health and Human Services was appalling. Where compassion and
urgency were called for, government officials offered indifference,
neglect, and outright hostility. The AIDS epidemic began while a
sharp scalpel was being taken to federal health and social welfare
programs, a coincidence with tragic consequences. By treating AIDS
as a series of state and local problems rather than as a national public
health disaster, the Reagan Administration guaranteed a fragmented
and inadequate response. Meanwhile, the epidemic spread.

By the late 1980s, the best that could be said was that the commitment of federal resources to AIDS had been cranked up and a formi-

236

dable research infrastructure was in place. But the FDA was languishing with ineffectual leadership and inadequate resources. ACTG researchers were still defending rigid trial designs that excluded many of the patients who most desperately needed experimental drugs. And pharmaceutical firms had priced many approved AIDS drugs out of patients' reach and were embroiled in licensing disputes that kept others from reaching the marketplace.

"There is a gap in the bureaucracy," said Martin Delaney. "There is no bureaucracy in this nation whose goal is to advocate on behalf of the needs of people with this disease. FDA's task is to keep unsafe or ineffective drugs out. NIH's task is to conduct the research. Whose task is to make sure that people get what they need? Nobody's."

In the early 1990s, conservative ideologues remain in power and still refuse to approach AIDS with the urgency they accorded previous health emergencies, such as Legionnaire's disease, because stigma still surrounds those principally affected. Vice-President Dan Quayle had been so little affected by a decade of AIDS that he could remark, with apparent sincerity, "Wouldn't it be wonderful if they found a cure for AIDS before Magic Johnson gets AIDS?" But the scientific and regulatory establishments have clearly intensified their efforts to identify and distribute AIDS drugs. With $1 billion in federal funds being spent on AIDS research every year, the changes within the FDA and other leading public health agencies have been dramatic.

The activist influence is unmistakable. "The rules have changed," said Jay Lipner. "It should now be understood that if you're a drug company, or you're the NIH and you're going to develop a drug, you're going to do it with the input of the people who are affected, and if you don't do it, you're going to get drowned."

The AIDS underground has been unprecedented. From 1985, when the smuggling networks were launched to bring ribavirin and isoprinosine into the United States from Mexico, until 1991, when clandestine chemists began manufacturing a pirated version of Hoffman–La Roche's ddC, activists challenged the law and public health policy without apology. Their message was clear: if scientists and bureaucrats refused to help, they would find ways to circumvent them. "AIDS patients have driven home to the U.S. medical and political establishment what enormous risks human beings in death's grip will take to gain relief or respite," said one *Wall Street Journal* editorial.

But in the long run, real influence would not come from building a separate system for obtaining drugs, but from becoming part of the decision-making process. And that is where the activists made enduring history.

The ganciclovir/foscarnet tragedy, personified in Terry Sutton, had been one of the FDA's most outstanding failures of imagination, a black mark it earned in the late 1980s. But by the time ddI was approved in 1991, the FDA had come a long way in its thinking about the relationship between patients' needs and the conduct of science.

Over the years, the agency made dramatic philosophical and procedural changes in response to AIDS. All AIDS drugs have been designated 1-A-A, a high-priority slot created specifically to put them at the head of the list for FDA review. Regulators are expected to review requests to begin human trials of new AIDS drugs within five days of receiving an application. Under the Sub-Part E regulations, they have also become more aggressive about offering guidance in the early stages of trial design to help sponsors avoid false starts. And, where drugs for life-threatening diseases are involved, the agency regularly reviews trial data in stages, and sometimes performs its own analyses. By beginning the review process before a drug company's licensing application is 100 percent complete, the FDA can shave months off its evaluation.

Meanwhile, Treatment IND and parallel track have markedly expanded patient access to promising drugs moving through the testing stages. When the accelerated drug approval process that was born on the heels of ddI is fully implemented, it too will help get new therapies to more patients. Taken together, the FDA has finally developed a set of flexible tools that allow it to distribute and approve safe and effective drugs more quickly. More significantly, it has proved willing to use those tools.

After a year adrift, the appointment of David Kessler as commissioner brought a sense of new possibilities to a beleaguered agency. He made law enforcement a top priority, and an agency that had been besieged by scandals began to straighten up its own act. In his first few months in office, the new commissioner took on the food industry, challenging misleading labels and false advertising. At first, the *Wall Street Journal* made some barbed remarks about Kessler's "food police," and ACT UP initially complained that he seemed more interested in food issues than in people with AIDS, but soon Kessler began to focus on drugs and helped turn the activists into allies. His challenge was clear, continuing efforts that were already under way: to push the FDA beyond its traditional mission of protecting consumers from unsafe or ineffective drugs. The additional mandate was to make safe and effective therapies available with appropriate haste. At the same time, the agency could not abandon all of its traditional standards. "The message is: Hurry up—carefully," warned one analyst. "More lives will be saved, in the end, by aiming accurately than by aiming early."

Tacrine, a potential treatment for Alzheimer's disease, was one of Kessler's first big challenges. It also became a litmus test of just how far the FDA was willing to go to expand access to unproven drugs.

The echo of AIDS was unmistakable. Once again, the agency was asked to approve a drug for a life-threatening disease for which no other therapies were available. Once again, advocates for an afflicted population were clamoring for the drug, despite some obvious limitations and apparent toxicities. And when an advisory committee voted against recommending approval, in March 1991, the *Wall Street Journal* once again attacked the FDA as an obstructionist regulator.

Shortly afterward, the FDA proposed that Warner-Lambert, tacrine's sponsor, run new studies. The company, which had been bitterly disappointed by the March decision, offered a possible compromise—it would sell tacrine as a Treatment IND, and conduct further studies, if the FDA guaranteed approval within a year, assuming the drug proved to be safe.

A few months later, the advisory committee met again to try to salvage the drug. Warner-Lambert's terms were not met. Instead, the committee recommended that the company be allowed to sell tacrine immediately while being required to conduct further research not merely to prove the drug's safety, but also to prove its effectiveness. That decision meant another three years of work before the company could sell tacrine at a high enough price to make a profit.

Warner-Lambert was chagrined at the setback, but others thought the decision was sound. A business-as-usual bureaucracy—the old FDA—might have looked at the available data, which was not terribly persuasive, and issued an unqualified rejection of tacrine. That decision would have denied desperate patients and their families the right to assume a reasonable risk for the prospect of some benefit. And it would have given the FDA's critics fresh ammunition to charge the agency with being as sluggish as ever.

On the other hand, an FDA too much in the pockets of the drug industry might have agreed to the Warner-Lambert approach, despite grave reservations about tacrine's therapeutic value. The agency would likely have been accused of pandering to patient desperation and allowing science to take a backseat to expediency. Consumer protectionists would surely have proclaimed the decision a step down the slippery and dangerous slope of deregulation.

But the new FDA found a third way, a zone of compromise that allowed patients to use a therapy of uncertain value while ensuring that credible scientific research continued. On December 2, 1991, the agency officially granted a Treatment IND for tacrine.

The FDA was shedding its image as a bureaucratic bottleneck for drugs, but the agency remains a troubled place. It is still burdened by layers of internal review and an inability to issue significant regulations without approval from overseers in the Department of Health and Human Services. Although Kessler has significantly reorganized the agency and infused it with a sense of optimism, the FDA desperately needs more staff and access to scientific expertise as sophisticated as what is available to the industry it regulates. A consolidated campus, or—at the very least—major reconstruction in facilities that have been described as "abysmal" would also be a pivotal step for bringing the FDA into the modern era. Without more generous congressional allocations, its ability to enforce the law and especially to pursue innovation is limited.

Moreover, the FDA's ability to move more aggressively to approve good drugs—without a rush to faulty judgments on the bad ones—will be tested over the next few years. Industry will surely continue to seek less regulation and easier access to new treatments. Consumer advocates will remember thalidomide and the scandals unfolding in 1992 of silicone breast implants and sleeping pills, in which manufacturers allegedly hid damning safety data, and resist any movement of the FDA too far from its role as protector of the public health. One mistake—one drug that proves too toxic after it is widely released—will likely set the regulatory pendulum swinging backward. Sam Broder warned of potentially "catastrophic consequences" if the FDA began moving too swiftly to release drugs. "I think we have to treat all of these drugs with respect," he said. "They are like open flames. You can light a path, you can get your way out of a tight spot with them, but there could be situations where you can get yourself very badly hurt. Open flames can burn you."

If the final verdict on the FDA must wait for the judgment of history, it is nonetheless clear that the agency in 1991 is very different from what it was at the birth of the AIDS epidemic. Mark Harrington called the agency "much more open and accessible than it ever used to be." During the agency's ddI deliberations, Martin Delaney praised it for becoming an "advocate for the public health," not just a gatekeeper. Kessler, in turn, gave the activists their due. "There's no question that they've had an enormous impact," he said. "There's been a change in the philosophy at the agency."

Far less progress has occurred in revamping reimbursement policies for experimental therapies. Although access to unapproved treatments can often prolong life or stave off serious symptoms, insurance companies typically refuse to pay for either the drugs or associated medical care.

The federal Health Care Financing Administration is one of the villains in this pecuniary reimbursement policy. HCFA decides what Medicare will pay for, setting an example that is typically followed by private health insurers. With medical costs soaring at the rate of ten to twelve percent a year, HCFA is under extraordinary pressure to curtail the use of unproven and expensive medicines. As a result, the agency has steadfastly refused to cover AIDS drugs dispensed under Treatment IND or parallel track, relegating access to those therapies only to the middle class or the wealthy. Moreover, as medical thinking evolves, physicians often prescribe drugs differently from the guidelines provided on the label. Yet it is common practice for HCFA and other insurance companies to deny reimbursement when a drug is prescribed for an unlabeled use.

HCFA's policies are inconsistent with its approach to cancer drugs.

In the mid-1970s, the FDA and the National Cancer Institute developed an informal classification known as Group C, to bring unproven cancer therapies to patients prior to FDA approval. Group C drugs are generally provided at no charge and HCFA reimburses for associated physician fees and laboratory charges.

There is no rationale for considering reimbursement on a disease-specific basis. A more coherent policy would cover investigational drugs for all grave illnesses when no other treatment is available. The double standard that rejects reimbursement for AIDS and other diseases while providing it for cancer is likely to stand only until it is challenged by lawsuits and activist vigor.

If ganciclovir was the FDA's Waterloo, NIAID's had been aerosolized pentamidine. Tony Fauci knew what had to be done to halt the killer disease, and he ran the nation's largest AIDS clinical trial system—but he could not get the study moving. NIAID's inability to test aerosolized pentamidine is a lasting source of shame.

Moreover, the record of the ACTG system remains unimpressive. Doctors on the frontlines of the epidemic still lack an adequate arsenal of drugs. And while the lifespan of people with AIDS has been extended as scientists have learned more about the course of the illness and found some new treatments, the disease remains almost inevitably fatal.

And yet, to his enduring credit, Tony Fauci helped make AIDS politics one of inclusion by giving the activists a meaningful voice in setting the nation's AIDS research agenda. Painful as the government's incompetent approach to pentamidine was, it did spawn a radical new approach to drug trials. Community-based testing now has federal funding and the stamp of approval from traditional researchers and has greatly increased the numbers of people, including minorities, women, and children, who can get experimental therapies at an early stage. A degree of cooperation and mutual respect between NIAID's research establishment and the activist community was ushered in with the new decade and Fauci was rewarded with "a pass through the sea of anger," according to Phil Hilts of the *New York Times*.

Despite the disappointing absence of scientific breakthroughs within the ACTG system, there have been meaningful shifts in its priorities. Having heard the complaints from Harrington, Eigo, and the rest, Fauci aggressively encouraged the trial sites to recruit more patients into existing studies targeted at opportunistic infections. By September 1991, 21 percent of all trial participants were testing drugs for AIDS-linked infections, up 300 percent from just two years earlier. Later that year, NIAID also funded a separate initiative to design OI drugs for AIDS.

As at the FDA, NIAID also pushed to identify surrogate markers, with the goal of speeding up and humanizing the whole system of drug research. For several years, activists and government statisticians have been working together to develop new ways to interpret complex trial data. The search for new methodologies is a highly technical process, but if it is successful it will allow researchers to loosen their entry criteria and broaden access to their trials.

Also in response to repeated cries from the activists, NIAID encouraged its clinical trial sites to attract a patient population more representative of the demographics of the AIDS epidemic. It used an attention-getting approach—money. Beginning in 1992, the federal dollars allocated to ACTG sites were linked directly to the diversity of trial enrollment.

And so there are signs of hope from the research establishment. Instead of expressing unrelenting hostility, men like Paul Boneberg, a San Francisco activist, are now willing to say, "When this plague is ended, it will be a joint victory of activists and scientists. Neither can do it alone, and that which divides us delays the day when the dying will end."

AIDS has also inspired a new wave of health activism. AIDS activists were not the first to lobby effectively on behalf of a specific disease. Historically, groups such as the American Heart Association, the Muscular Dystrophy Foundation, and the American Cancer Society amassed considerable financial resources and a great deal of political clout. But there was an essential difference in their approach: leading scientists and philanthropists always directed their research; the patient population never led the charge toward clinical advances.

Even the quest for an effective polio vaccine, which relied heavily on the initiatives of volunteers, was not really a grassroots effort. The voluntary gifts of time and money from thousands of individual citizens dwarfed the support from the federal government, but always the direction came from the top.

AIDS changed the picture, and now its lessons are being replayed across the country. From breast cancer to schizophrenia, constituent groups have discovered that by speaking knowledgeably, and sometimes by shouting loudly, they can shake the medical establishment to its foundations. Like their AIDS activist counterparts, they have begun to clamor for a more urgent approach to clinical research and drug approval, for the right to make informed choices about the risks they will accept, and for better access to care. They are also finding common cause with one another; coalition-building is the name of the game in the 1990s.

Susan Love is an example of the new breed of activists. Love, a well-known breast cancer physician who leads a national coalition of advocacy groups, clearly borrowed ACT UP phrasing when she declared in a Washington speech: "No more politeness. We are not going to be cheerleaders and fundraisers for the same old system. We need to tell the truth to women. Our intention is to become experts about the breast cancer establishment. We need to demand a place in the design of trials, and hold researchers accountable for women's lives."

Activist language is also evident in the Statement of Purpose of the Cancer Patient Action Alliance (CAN ACT). The New York–based group of cancer patients and their advocates called the FDA's insistence on protracted clinical trials "unreasonable and capricious" when drugs had been approved abroad. CAN ACT also called for greater access to drugs available in Europe, Canada, and Asia, and criticized the health insurance industry for "denying reimbursement to cancer patients for treatment involving innovative therapy."

Drug pricing is another issue in which patient advocates found common ground. Historically, the right to determine drug prices has belonged to the pharmaceutical industry. Not so with AIDS.

The activists' willingness to battle corporate profiteers became a model for schizophrenia patients and their advocates in 1990, when Sandoz priced a year's therapy with clozapine, a new antipsychotic drug to control schizophrenia, at an outrageous $9,000. It was more than four times what the drug was selling for in Europe, mostly because Sandoz insisted that patients also purchase an expensive blood-monitoring system, ostensibly to guard against potential drug toxicities. The Sandoz policy: "No blood, no drug." The real motivation was protecting profit margins by reducing its liability risk.

The high price of clozapine meant that mentally ill patients were being gouged. More than twenty states joined in a lawsuit against the Swiss-based manufacturer, claiming the company could not legally require the drug and the monitoring system to be purchased as a package. The antitrust subcommittee of the Senate's Judiciary Committee scheduled hearings on the subject. In the face of mounting political pressures, Sandoz backed down and dropped its monitoring requirement. The price fell by almost half.

It is probably not too far a stretch to argue that if Peter Staley and his friends had not invaded Burroughs Wellcome's headquarters or the New York Stock Exchange to protest the price of AZT . . . if the price Lyphomed slapped on pentamidine had gone unquestioned . . . if Derek Hodel had not directed the New York buyers' club to import pentamidine from England so that patients could buy it more cheaply . . . quite possibly, the price of clozapine would never have been challenged.

AIDS has shown that patients could make a difference.

Still, with an estimated 40,000 new HIV infections occurring in the United States every year, and an AIDS caseload above 200,000 by January 1992, there is little cause for rejoicing. Without an effective treatment or a vaccine, the future looks bleak for those who are infected. Despite reports that suggest the epidemic has peaked in North America, the social fabric in our cities continues to unravel as the twin tragedies of AIDS and drug abuse take their toll. And in parts of the underdeveloped world, the devastation is almost unfathomable: Between *30* and *40 million* people around the globe are expected to be infected by the end of the decade.

A drug to stop HIV in its tracks is nowhere on the horizon, and years of testing lie ahead before a vaccine is likely to become available. "I think everybody is looking for the magic bullet and I think we need to keep searching for it," said Sam Broder. "But we have got to make sure that people remember there are limits to what these drugs can do. It is exceedingly unlikely that in the near future we are going to have any drug that doesn't have some side effects."

Instead, Broder, like most other scientific experts, hopes that HIV infection can someday be treated as a manageable chronic disease. "I think the model we will eventually have for it is high blood pressure," he said. "If you catch it early enough, it's possible with the appropriate medical intervention to make a dramatic impact."

Neither the promise of future breakthroughs nor the greater efficiencies in the drug approval process have been enough to make Larry Kramer optimistic. Nor is he sanguine about the real value of an activist presence at the policy table. His pleas for a "Manhattan project" against AIDS—an effort to match the commitment of scientific energies poured into the construction of the atomic bomb—have been ignored. His call for terrorism at the San Francisco AIDS conference was harshly criticized.

"I'm convinced that the war has been lost. There's no way the system is going to be able to respond," a disheartened Kramer said as the new decade began. "The nature of bureaucracy is such that until Bush puts someone in charge, a cure could be found tomorrow and there would be no way to push it through the thick bureaucracy."

Not everyone shares that dark outlook. In a rebuttal to Kramer, Paul Boneberg wrote, "The scientists and physicians are our allies. . . . We are working with some of the best medical minds alive in the world, and to blame them for not defeating AIDS more quickly is to shoot the messenger who brings bad news."

The Kramer-Boneberg debate, like the judgment on AIDS drug development in general, comes down to a question of perspective. Clearly, the nation's bureaucratic and political responses to the epidemic were at times disgraceful. And yet it is equally certain that biomedical science has made tremendous strides in understanding AIDS over the past ten years. It is also clear that the federal regulatory agencies pledged to protect the public health have slowly, painstakingly, found ways to change.

For now, the story of AIDS drug development remains a struggle between those who have all the time in the world and those for whom time is running out. But it also remains a story of hope—a hope that holds steadfast against the odds.

Appendix A

MILESTONES IN AIDS DRUG DEVELOPMENT

1931
- The Food and Drug Administration, successor to the Bureau of Chemistry and the Food, Drug and Insecticide Administration, is organized to monitor the nation's food supply and the drug industry.

1938
- Soon after Elixir Sulfanilamide kills 100 patients, the Food, Drug and Cosmetic Act is passed, making it illegal to market a drug until it has been proven safe.

1949
- The Nuremberg Code, defining the structure of an ethical experiment on human beings, is promulgated in the wake of revelations about Nazi research.

OCTOBER 1962
- Spurred partially by the thalidomide tragedy, the Kefauver Amendments to the Food, Drug and Cosmetic Act are passed, requiring that drugs prove not only safe, but effective.

1964
- Jerome Horwitz, a cancer researcher in Detroit, synthesizes AZT for the first time. The drug proves to have little value and is shelved.

1974
- Wolfram Ostergag, a researcher at the Max Planck Institute in Germany, publishes findings that show AZT to be effective against animal retroviruses.

JUNE 1981
- The Centers for Disease Control publishes an article in *Morbidity and Mortality Weekly Report* about the unusual occurrence of *Pneumocystis*

carinii pneumonia (PCP) in five gay men from Los Angeles. It is the first published hint of a looming epidemic.

JULY 1981
• The *New York Times* describes the mysterious increase in Kaposi's sarcoma among homosexuals. The rare cancer, traditionally seen in older Italian and Jewish men, is soon nicknamed "gay cancer."

JANUARY 1982
• Total reported AIDS cases: 394. Death toll: 163.

JUNE 1982
• The Gay Men's Health Crisis is incorporated under New York State law to provide services and advocate for public policies for people with AIDS.

SEPTEMBER 1982
• The Centers for Disease Control declares a new epidemic and coins the name acquired immune deficiency syndrome, or AIDS.

JANUARY 1983
• Total reported AIDS cases: 1,501. Death toll: 612.
• The Orphan Drug Act is signed into law providing exclusive marketing rights, tax breaks and other lucrative incentives to push drug companies into developing therapies for rare diseases.

MAY 1983
• Twelve French scientists publish their findings on a new human retrovirus, isolated from Frédéric Brugière, a Parisian fashion designer. Eventually this new virus is identified as human immunodeficiency virus—HIV.

JANUARY 1984
• Total reported AIDS cases: 4,489. Death toll: 2,081.

APRIL 1984
• Secretary of Health and Human Services Margaret Heckler announces the discovery of the virus believed to cause AIDS. Robert Gallo of the National Cancer Institute and Luc Montagnier of the Pasteur Institute in Paris launch a seven-year battle over credit for the discovery.

MAY 1984
• FDA gives Syntex permission to distribute ganciclovir, which can halt cytomegalovirus retinitis and prevent blindness, on a compassionate-use basis.

OCTOBER 1984

- Sam Broder, director of the National Cancer Institute (NCI), meets with Burroughs Wellcome and tries to prod it into AIDS research. Soon the company begins sending chemical compounds to NCI for screening.
- Lyphomed receives FDA approval to market injectable pentamidine, designed to treat or prevent the fatal *Pneumocystis carinii* pneumonia.
- Lyphomed receives an orphan drug designation for injectable pentamidine.

JANUARY 1985

- Total reported AIDS cases: 10,502. Death toll: 5,440.
- The first drug-smuggling operation begins. Mexico is the source, and the targets are ribavirin, a multipurpose antiviral drug believed effective against HIV, and isoprinosine, which appears to boost the immune system.
- Ethigen, then called Praxis Pharmaceuticals, goes public. AL-721, lipids derived from egg yolks, are its only product, and stock shares sell at $1.25.

FEBRUARY 1985

- Hiroaki Mitsuya, a researcher in Sam Broder's National Cancer Institute laboratory, demonstrates AZT's effectiveness against HIV in the test tube for the first time. Duke University scientists confirm the finding.

MARCH 1985

- The FDA licenses a test to protect the nation's blood supply against HIV by screening for antibodies.
- The County Community Consortium, which becomes a locus of community-based drug testing, is founded in San Francisco.
- Burroughs Wellcome files for its British patent on AZT.

SPRING 1985

- Preparation begins on the first scientific abstract to document AZT's activity against the AIDS virus for the first time. Correspondence between Sam Broder and Sandra Lehrman, a senior researcher at Burroughs Wellcome, is evidence of close collaboration.

MAY 1985

- U.S. Customs begins to confiscate ribavirin and isoprinosine at the Mexican border.

JUNE 1985

- Burroughs Wellcome files an investigational new drug (IND) application with the FDA that allows AZT to be tested in humans.

JULY 1985

• A Boston furniture salesman becomes the first person to take AZT, and Phase I trials begin at NCI and Duke. Eschewing the usual responsibilities of a corporate partner, Burroughs Wellcome refuses to analyze patient blood samples, fearing contamination from the AIDS virus. The company is nonetheless granted an orphan drug designation for AZT.

SEPTEMBER 1985

• The American Foundation for AIDS Research (AmFAR) is founded by Mathilde Krim and Michael Gottlieb when the AIDS Medical Foundation of New York merges with the National AIDS Research Foundation of Los Angeles.
• Project Inform is founded by Martin Delaney and others.
• Burroughs Wellcome files for an American patent on AZT. In its patent application, it makes broad claims for the value of the drug and does not mention the contributions of others in the development process. This may have been a breach of the legal obligation to name all coinventors, as well as a breach of the "duty of candor."

NOVEMBER 1985

• Robert Gallo's letter reporting that AL-721 might inhibit HIV is published in the *New England Journal of Medicine*. The stock of Ethigen, which owns the AL-721 patent, more than triples in price to four dollars a share.

JANUARY 1986

• Total reported AIDS cases: 21,780. Death toll: 12,097.
• The U.S. Patent and Trademark Office rejects Burroughs Wellcome's first patent application on AZT, claiming the company had failed to show that AZT had "utility" against the virus.

FEBRUARY 1986

• Phase II trials of AZT begin, financed by Burroughs Wellcome and run at NCI and Duke University.

MARCH 1986

• Hiroaki Mitsuya and Sam Broder publish findings indicating that ddI, a cousin of AZT, inhibits replication of the AIDS virus in the test tube.
• Robert Yarchoan, Sam Broder, Hiroaki Mitsuya, and other National Cancer Institute and Burroughs Wellcome researchers publish their AZT Phase I trial results in the British medical journal *The Lancet*.

JUNE 1986

• The National Institute for Allergy and Infectious Diseases (NIAID) establishes the first government AIDS research program, the AIDS Treatment Evaluation Units, the predecessor to the AIDS Clinical Trial Group.

SUMMER 1986
- Don Abrams, a researcher at San Francisco General Hospital, learns from Japanese scientist Ryuji Ueno that dextran sulfate may be effective against the AIDS virus and decides to test it.

SEPTEMBER 1986
- Placebo-controlled Phase II trials demonstrate AZT's effectiveness. The trial is halted so that all participants can get the drug.

DECEMBER 1986
- Burroughs Wellcome files a New Drug Application with the FDA, asking for permission to market AZT.

WINTER 1987
- Don Abrams begins a Phase I trial of dextran sulfate.

JANUARY 1987
- Total reported AIDS cases: 40,134. Death toll: 23,511.
- The first issue of *AIDS Treatment News* is published by John James to provide patients with treatment information about both approved and unapproved drugs.

FEBRUARY 1987
- A NIAID subcommittee calls aerosolized pentamidine a high-priority drug and urges that it be tested for its value against PCP in government trials.

MARCH 1987
- The FDA proposes the Treatment IND initiative, which will permit the sale of promising but unapproved drugs. Critics are concerned that drugs need not prove they are effective before being released.
- Syntex receives a patent for ganciclovir.
- Burroughs Wellcome receives FDA approval to market AZT. Shortly afterward, the company announces AZT will cost patients $10,000 a year, and Congressman Henry Waxman holds hearings to probe the reasons for its high cost.
- The AIDS Coalition to Unleash Power (ACT UP) is born in the basement of a Greenwich Village community center. Its first demonstration is staged on Wall Street to protest the price of AZT.
- An underground business partnership is formed in New York to develop

and distribute AL-721. Although interest wanes in AL-721, the partnership evolves into one of the nation's first buyers' clubs.

MAY 1987
- Michael Callen, activist and long-term AIDS survivor, meets with Tony Fauci, director of NIAID, to ask for guidelines advising local physicians to give their patients medication to prevent PCP. Fauci says no.
- Final Treatment IND regulations are published in the *Federal Register*.
- The Community Research Initiative, formed to run community-based trials, opens for business in New York City.

JULY 1987
- San Francisco's County Community Consortium begins testing aerosolized pentamidine.
- Protocol 019, designed to test the value of AZT in asymptomatic people infected with HIV, is launched by Paul Volberding of San Francisco General Hospital.

AUGUST 1987
- Lyphomed hikes the price of aerosolized pentamidine to $99.45, quadrupling the cost in just three years.
- Worldwide sales of AZT reach $25 million.

FALL 1987
- Head smuggler James Corti, soon to be known as "Dextran Man," devises an underground network to import dextran sulfate from Japan.

OCTOBER 1987
- Fisons receives orphan drug designation for its version of aerosolized pentamidine.
- An advisory committee says the FDA should reject Syntex's application to market ganciclovir, citing inadequate data. Patients and their physicians are outraged, since almost everyone believes the drug prevents blindness.

JANUARY 1988
- Total reported AIDS cases: 67,450. Death toll: 38,858.
- A NIAID advisory committee issues a report criticizing the AIDS Treatment Evaluation Units, NIAID's first attempt to create an AIDS research system.
- Lyphomed receives orphan drug designation for its version of aerosolized pentamidine.
- The federal government grants Bristol-Myers the rights to develop and ultimately market ddI.

February 1988

- Burroughs Wellcome's American patent application for AZT is approved and is issued patent number 4,724,232.
- Trimetrexate, which has proven effective against PCP, becomes the first AIDS drug awarded Treatment IND status. The terms under which the FDA allows its distribution enrage activists.

March 1988

- Protocol 045, a placebo-controlled immunoglobulin trial designed to stave off bacterial infections in children, begins. The study horrifies some observers because it subjects HIV-infected children to undue discomfort without hope of gain.
- NIAID enrolls its first patient in its aerosolized pentamidine trial, one year after community groups begin testing the drug.

Spring 1988

- In response to harsh criticism, NIAID restructures its AIDS research program and the AIDS Clinical Trial Group (ACTG) is born.
- The Japanese shut down the dextran sulfate pipeline, and Americans lose access to the drug.

June 1988

- The Presidential Commission on the HIV Epidemic issues its final report, attacking the lack of federal leadership and calling for more resources and prevention efforts, better patient management, and enhanced research.
- Peter Staley organizes a sit-in at Kowa Pharmaceuticals, the manufacturer of dextran sulfate. Eleven activists occupy Kowa's New York office and demand the right to buy the drug in Japan.

July 1988

- FDA Commissioner Frank Young announces a revised personal-use import policy that will allow small quantities of unapproved drugs to be carried or mailed across international borders. He is both praised and mocked for his efforts.

Summer 1988

- ACTG Protocol 071, designed to test ganciclovir in patients with peripheral retinitis, is launched in the hopes of salvaging the drug. Almost no one enrolls.
- The FDA agrees to expand the terms of its controversial trimetrexate Treatment IND.
- In a Phase I study at the National Cancer Institute, ddI is administered to AIDS patients for the first time.

AUGUST 1988
- Worldwide sales of AZT reach $183 million.

OCTOBER 1988
- Carrying placards reading "I Died on Placebo" and "Rest in Peace, Killed by the FDA," ACT UP demonstrates at FDA headquarters in Rockville, Maryland, to focus attention on the sluggish pace of drug approvals.
- The FDA announces innovations, known as the Sub-Part E regulations and patterned after the approach used to evaluate AZT, designed to speed the assessment of drugs for life-threatening diseases.

NOVEMBER 1988
- The FDA gives ganciclovir Treatment IND status for use against cytomegalovirus retinitis, but cancels the broader compassionate-use program that got the drug to most patients who needed it.

JANUARY 1989
- Total reported AIDS cases: 100,431. Death toll: 58,360.
- NIAID requests proposals to fund community-based research programs, underscoring the legitimacy of a concept it once called too novel.
- Michael McGrath of San Francisco General Hospital, Hin-Wing Yeung of the Chinese University of Hong Kong, and two GeneLabs researchers share the patent for GLQ-223, a purified version of Compound Q.
- Tony Fauci meets Terry Sutton and gains new insight into the human cost of bureaucratic decisions. He decides to lobby for the approval of ganciclovir.
- Demonstrators block access across the Golden Gate Bridge in San Francisco to dramatize the need for more AIDS drugs. Activist Terry Sutton is jailed.

FEBRUARY 1989
- Aerosolized pentamidine is awarded Treatment IND status by the FDA.

MARCH 1989
- The PWA Health Group begins to import fluconazole, used to treat cryptococcal meningitis, an inflammation of the brain and nervous system. It is the first time the buyers' club brings prescription drugs across international borders.

APRIL 1989
- Terry Sutton dies without getting the chance to try foscarnet.
- ACT UP invades Burroughs Wellcome's North Carolina headquarters to protest the high price of AZT.

- AmFAR announces $1.4 million in grants to stimulate community-based research.

MAY 1989
- Project Inform launches underground trials of Compound Q in San Francisco, New York, Los Angeles, and Fort Lauderdale, but fails to comply with many conventions of drug research.

JUNE 1989
- The Fifth International AIDS Conference is held in Montreal. Tony Fauci and Larry Kramer are reconciled, the New York buyers' club learns it can buy cheap pentamidine abroad, and Sam Broder talks enthusiastically about ddI.
- Lyphomed receives FDA approval to market aerosolized pentamidine, based largely on data generated by community-based trials.
- Syntex receives FDA approval to market ganciclovir.
- Tony Fauci proposes the parallel-track initiative, designed to speed access to experimental drugs while allowing formal trials to continue.
- Robert Parr dies on the underground Compound Q trial, and the veil of secrecy is stripped away.
- Erythropoietin (EPO), developed for AIDS-related anemias, becomes the fourth AIDS drug to receive Treatment IND status.
- Under pressure from activists, NIAID launches a new initiative to expand opportunistic infection research.
- The National Institutes of Health drafts conflict-of-interest guidelines that generate consternation among ACTG researchers.

JULY 1989
- Sam Broder's Phase I study of ddI is published, and the results are promising.

AUGUST 1989
- Protocol 019 indicates that AZT slows progression to AIDS among asymptomatic individuals with HIV infection. The trial is halted so all participants can get the drug.
- Worldwide sales of AZT reach $408 million, and a lead editorial in the *New York Times* calls the price of AZT "astoundingly high."
- An FDA advisory committee holds hearings on parallel track, attended by most of the major players on the AIDS drug scene. A parallel-track working group, assembled to flesh out Fauci's original proposal, holds its first meeting shortly afterward.
- Carl Peck of the FDA asks Martin Delaney to halt the underground

Compound Q study, but invites him to present accumulated data to the agency.

- Scott Scheaffer dies after participating in the New York arm of the Compound Q trial.

SEPTEMBER 1989

- Treatment IND status is given to ddI by the FDA.
- Fujisawa, a Japanese pharmaceutical firm, takes control of Lyphomed, the manufacturer of pentamidine. John Kapoor, the board chairman of Lyphomed, pockets $133 million as a result of the sale.
- ACT UP invades the New York Stock Exchange to protest the price of AZT. Activist foghorns drown out the opening trading bell.
- The PWA Health Group begins importing pentamidine from England. For the first time the buyers' club has gone overseas not to obtain unapproved drugs but to save patients' money.
- T. E. Haigler, then president of Burroughs Wellcome, claims the lion's share of the credit for the AZT discovery in a letter published in the *New York Times*. Broder is inflamed. AIDS activist groups begin exploring a possible challenge to the AZT patent with Congressman Ted Weiss.

OCTOBER 1989

- DdI is made available on an expanded-access basis and formal Phase II ACTG clinical trials begin eight days afterward; the parallel-track initiative is launched.
- NIAID announces the winners of its community-based research awards program. The Community Research Initiative, one of the pioneers of the concept, is not on the winner's list and protests noisily.
- ACTG researchers announce that its data analysis functions will be transferred from the Research Triangle Institute in North Carolina to the Harvard School of Public Health—and new trials will be postponed until the transfer is complete.
- AZT is awarded Treatment IND status for pediatric AIDS.
- In a rebuttal to T. E. Haigler, Sam Broder and others at NCI and Duke University reaffirm their contributions to the development of AZT.
- Martin Delaney meets with the FDA to present data from the underground Compound Q study. Instead of slapping his wrist, the agency tells him the terms under which he can continue the research.
- Refusing to take no for an answer, ACT UP representatives crash a meeting of ACTG researchers.

DECEMBER 1989

- Frank Young is removed from his post as FDA Commissioner largely in

response to the generic-drug scandal, and is given a lesser position else-where in the Department of Health and Human Services.
- ACT UP stages a protest inside St. Patrick's Cathedral, and Tom Keane scandalizes the church by crumbling a communion wafer on the floor.
- The Community Constituency Working Group, established to provide consumer input into the ACTG process, meets for the first time.
- Following angry protests, the National Institutes of Health shelves its conflict-of-interest guidelines for researchers.

1990
- At Sam Broder's insistence, the National Institutes of Health hires outside counsel to investigate the legitimacy of Burroughs Wellcome's patent. Counsel determines there are grounds for a challenge.

JANUARY 1990
- Total reported AIDS cases: 137,310. Death toll: 83,681.
- Pfizer receives FDA approval to market fluconazole for cryptococcal meningitis.

FEBRUARY 1990
- ACT UP "zaps" Astra, demanding expanded access to foscarnet.

MARCH 1990
- The FDA approves Project Inform's new study design for further Compound Q trials.
- Louis Sullivan appoints the Edwards Committee, named for Charles Edwards, chief executive officer of Scripps Clinic and Research Foundation and a former FDA Commissioner, to examine the shortcomings and potential of the FDA.

APRIL 1990
- Results of Protocol 019, showing the value of AZT in early intervention, are published in the *New England Journal of Medicine* almost three years after the trial began, and eight months after preliminary findings were released at a press conference.

MAY 1990
- Burroughs Wellcome receives FDA approval to market AZT for pediatric AIDS.
- At an ACTG meeting, ACT UP distributes its critique of the government's clinical trial system to researchers and the press.
- The parallel-track proposal is published in the *Federal Register* almost a year after the concept was put forward by Tony Fauci.

- Underscoring its shift of focus from the drug approval process to the drug testing process, ACT UP stages a demonstration on the campus of the National Institutes of Health.

JUNE 1990

- The Sixth International AIDS Conference is held in San Francisco. Martin Delaney and Arnold Relman, then editor-in-chief of the *New England Journal of Medicine,* clash over the underground Compound Q trial.

SUMMER 1990

- Tony Fauci imposes financial disclosure requirements on ACTG researchers to safeguard against conflicts of interest.

AUGUST 1990

- The Lasagna Committee, named for Louis Lasagna, dean of Tufts Medical School, issues its final report and calls for expediting drug approvals, especially where life-threatening diseases are involved.
- NIAID announces $2.8 million in first-year funding for six teams of scientists to design drugs targeted at AIDS-related opportunistic infections.
- Worldwide sales of AZT reach $696 million.

SEPTEMBER 1990

- Results of the County Community Consortium's aerosolized pentamidine trials are published in the *New England Journal of Medicine,* one year after the drug was approved.
- Astra submits its application to market foscarnet, and begins distributing the drug on a compassionate-use basis, years after the first request for expanded access was made.

OCTOBER 1990

- David A. Kessler's nomination as new FDA Commissioner is approved by the United States Senate in the waning hours of its fall session.

NOVEMBER 1990

- NIAID announces that every ACTG committee will have constituent representation, a long-standing activist goal.
- Despite a unanimous vote in Congress, George Bush kills reform of the Orphan Drug Act with a pocket veto. The reforms would have sharply restricted the financial incentives to rare-drug development once more than 200,000 patients were diagnosed with a disease. Lyphomed has lobbied hard for the veto.

DECEMBER 1990

- Apotex and Novopharm, two small Canadian drug companies, file a court challenge to Burroughs Wellcome's exclusive AZT patent.

- Ellen Cooper resigns her position as director of the FDA's ant⸢
sion, citing the impossible pressures of the job.

JANUARY 1991
- Total reported AIDS cases: 171,574. Death toll: 108,120.

MARCH 1991
- Public Citizen files a lawsuit in U.S. District Court seeking to invalida⸢
Burroughs Wellcome's AZT patent.
- A Phase II trial begins on Peptide T, five years after the antiviral drug was
invented. The delays reflect a combination of interinstitutional rivalry,
professional ego, and possible conflicts of interest.

APRIL 1991
- Barr Laboratories, a New York–based generic-drug manufacturer, asks
the FDA for permission to manufacture and sell its version of AZT for the
treatment of HIV disease.

MAY 1991
- Burroughs Wellcome files suit against Barr Laboratories in U.S. District
Court for infringing on six of its AZT patents. Barr countersues soon
afterward, demanding that the National Institutes of Health be named
coinventor of the patent.
- The Edwards Committee issues its final report on the FDA and says the
agency is "under stress." It recommends that drugs for life-threatening
diseases be made available as quickly as possible when there are no
therapeutic alternatives.
- Treatment IND status is awarded to ddC, an antiviral drug in the same
family as AZT and ddI.

JUNE 1991
- The Seventh International AIDS Conference is held in Florence, Italy.
Thirteen vaccines are in various stages of human testing around the world,
and the subject of vaccine development dominates conference discussions.

JULY 1991
- The National Institutes of Health grants a conditional marketing license
for AZT to Barr Laboratories, provided the company prevails in its lawsuit
challenging Burroughs Wellcome's patent.

AUGUST 1991
- Worldwide sales of AZT top $1 billion.

SEPTEMBER 1991
- Astra receives FDA approval to market foscarnet, used to treat AIDS

with cytomegalovirus retinitis. The drug is priced at $21,000 per

ᴇʀ 1991

stol-Myers receives FDA approval to market ddI for adult and pediat-
ᴄ patients with advanced HIV disease. The drug is labeled for use by
patients who cannot tolerate AZT or whose condition has deteriorated
while on the drug. The annual price of ddI is $1,745 per year.

NOVEMBER 1991
• Senators Nancy Landon Kassebaum and Howard Metzenbaum introduce
Orphan Drug Act reform legislation to rescind a company's exclusive
marketing rights once drug sales top $200 million.

JANUARY 1992
• Total reported AIDS cases: 206,392. Death toll: 133,232.

APRIL 1992
• FDA regulations published in the Federal Register spell out the terms of
the parallel track distribution and accelerated approval. Parallel track
provides wider access to experimental drugs while formal trials continue;
accelerated approval allows drugs to be marketed on the basis of preliminary data but requires them to be pulled quickly from pharmacy shelves
if they prove ineffective.

MAY 1992
• In attempts to assuage activist protests, Astra drops the price of foscarnet
by 15 percent.

JUNE 1992
• Hoffman LaRoche receives FDA approval to market ddC as an antiviral
drug in combination with AZT. Like ddI, it is released under the fast-track,
accelerated approval system.
• In a bizarre twist of allegiances, Peter Staley, of ACT UP/New York
brokers a million dollar gift from Burroughs Wellcome to support
community-based AIDS research.

AUGUST 1992
• Worldwide sales of AZT reach $1.4 billion.

OCTOBER 1992
• Total reported AIDS cases: 242,146. Death toll: 160,372.

Appendix B

How a Clinical Trial Is Designed

THE FIRST KNOWN CLINICAL TRIAL took place on an oceangoing vessel in 1747. Twelve sailors were afflicted with scurvy, long the bane of a seafaring man's life. James Lind, a British naval surgeon, decided to experiment on the ailing mariners by offering them six different treatment regimens: cider, elixir of vitriol, vinegar, seawater, nutmeg, and citrus fruit. Within a few days, the men on a daily dose of two oranges and a lemon were declared fit for duty. Naval officials subsequently included limes with meal rations, so the trial had its desired outcome (and also gave the British seaman the nickname "Limey").

The system for testing new drugs today is presumably more sophisticated and certainly is more cumbersome than it was in the age of scurvy, but the broad concept remains much the same: patients suffering from the same ailment are given different substances, or the same substance at differing doses, so that scientists can compare results and identify effective treatments. Well-designed, carefully executed clinical trials show physicians whether a drug works and in what doses it should be prescribed, and alert them to potential side effects.

Since the Kefauver Amendments to the Food, Drug and Cosmetic Act were passed in 1962, the process for testing new drugs has looked like this:

THE PRE-CLINICAL STAGE

The pre-clinical stage, usually lasting about eighteen months, begins after a promising drug is identified in the test tube and lasts until animal tests have been completed. Typically, 10 percent of the substances screened in these early studies show some potential. Of, say, 2,000 compounds, just 200 will

261

...ising. Commercial and scientific considerations then dictate which
...ually get tested in humans; perhaps 20 of the 200 will make the cut.

INVESTIGATIONAL NEW DRUG

... be tested in humans, a drug requires a sponsor—usually a pharmaceuti-
al company or an academic or government researcher—who must submit
an investigational new drug (IND) application to the FDA. (In 1990, the
FDA received 316 IND applications from industry and 1,334 sponsored by
academic investigators.) After a slow start, when only a handful of INDs
were filed for AIDS drugs, the numbers jumped sharply. By the end of 1991,
more than 500 AIDS-related clinical studies were under way.

The IND applications are mammoth, sometimes running as long as 1,250
pages. Each one provides data from test-tube and animal experiments, as
well as from any human trials that may have been conducted abroad. And
it provides a script, known as a **protocol**, that spells out the minutiae of future
human trials. A well-designed trial includes a purpose, criteria for participation, how long it is to last, the controls to be used, the number of subjects,
the relative risk/benefit ratio, the conditions under which an ailing patient
is to be removed from a study, and the statistical methods proposed to
evaluate the findings. The objective of the protocol is to ensure that it will
generate valid data.

Most trials are also **controlled** and **randomized**. That is, they are designed
so that one group of patients can be compared against another group, with
subjects assigned to either the treatment or the control arm of the study in
some random manner. Many different types of controls are possible. The
controversial placebo-controlled trial, in which some people get the test drug
while others are given an inert substance, has traditionally been viewed as
the fastest and most scientifically precise way to determine whether a particular effect is produced by an experimental drug or by some other variable,
including pure chance. Other controls include comparing an experimental
drug at two different doses or comparing it against an effective therapy
already in general use.

Controlled trials may also be **blind** or **double-blind**. In a blind study, the
patient does not know what he or she is taking; in a double-blind study,
neither patient nor researcher is privy to that information. Randomized,
controlled, and blinded studies are considered ethical only when there is
genuine doubt as to which of two alternatives is safer and more effective.

Traditionally, researchers test new drugs on fairly homogeneous popula-

tions. By recruiting individuals who are generally within the same a
and of the same sex and who have similar medical histories, research
be more certain that differing trial results stem from the drug being
rather than from extraneous factors. On the surface it seems justifiable,
the consequence is that women and minority populations have been s
tematically underrepresented in clinical trials. AIDS drugs, for exampl
have been tested primarily on white gay males, a fact that has been a major
sore spot among patient advocates.

Another important element of the protocol is the **trial endpoint**—in other
words, what markers will be used to determine whether a drug is effective.
For AIDS, death and increased survival time have long been the standards
of measurement. But with AZT in widespread use and effective therapies
available to prevent or delay killer pneumonia, most people with AIDS are
living longer. That means it can be years before scientists know whether a
new drug actually extends life, making body counts unethical. Where possible, scientists now define "surrogate endpoints," such as the health of the
immune system or the level of viral activity in the blood, in order to reduce
the time necessary to measure a drug's effectiveness. By 1991 the FDA had
demonstrated its willingness to accept surrogate markers as evidence of drug
efficacy.

Unless the FDA notifies the sponsor to the contrary, a drug may be tested
in humans thirty days after an IND is submitted. Pharmaceutical sponsors
do not generally run their own trials. Instead, they contract with universities,
teaching hospitals, or, in the case of AIDS, the growing number of community-based organizations equipped to test new drugs. The National Institutes
of Health sponsors some of its own drug trials through an in-house research
program, and also oversees the huge AIDS Clinical Trial Group program at
academic medical centers and community agencies across the country.

Whenever human subjects are involved in testing drugs, trial design must
be approved by a local **Institutional Review Board.** Most research centers
have their own IRBs, whose members review protocols, critique informed-
consent forms, monitor trial ethics, and make certain that all participants
understand the trial goals and are appropriately protected.

THE THREE PHASES OF DRUG TESTING

Under the Kefauver Amendments, the FDA required for the first time that
data from "adequate and well-controlled trials" be used to determine a
drug's effectiveness. To meet that one-sentence legislative mandate, a

sometimes ponderous process has evolved to move a drug from
,ational status to approval. Until the dawn of the AIDS epidemic, that
1 remained largely intact.

common practice, although not by law, clinical trials are conducted in
.ee phases so that a drug is tested on increasingly larger populations as
-ore information becomes known about safety and efficacy. About 20 per-
:ent of the drugs that enter the first phase of human testing are ultimately
approved for marketing; the rest drop out along the way because they prove
to be unsafe, ineffective, or commercially impractical.

Phase I tests focus on safety, generally take less than a year, and involve
relatively few patients. Trials at this stage attempt to determine a drug's
toxicity and mode of absorption, how the drug is eliminated from the body,
the best method of administration, and the safest dosage. Because of the
urgency of finding new therapies for AIDS, researchers have also tried to
extract some efficacy data from Phase I studies.

Phase II trials involve a limited number of patients—generally fewer than
200—and typically take two years. At this stage, investigators want to determine a drug's efficacy, confirm its safety, pinpoint appropriate dosage levels
more precisely, and compare it to similar drugs. In the wake of the Kefauver
Amendments, the Food and Drug Administration required controls of some
sort so that the cleanest possible data possible could be generated. Much of
the pressure to speed access to AIDS drugs has been directed at Phase II
trials.

In **Phase III,** several thousand patients may be involved in controlled
studies that confirm and elaborate on all the information gathered in Phase
II. These trials, which usually take between one and three years, emphasize
long-term safety and efficacy. More than 95 percent of the drugs that reach
Phase III trials are eventually approved for marketing.

THE NEW DRUG APPLICATION

After Phase III is completed, the drug's sponsor analyzes its data and submits a New Drug Application (NDA) to the FDA. A massive amount of
information is required for an NDA; the summary itself often runs 200 pages
or more, and the total application may contain thousands of pages of documentation.

Once the FDA receives an NDA, the clock begins to tick. By law, the FDA
has just 180 days to reject or approve an application. In practice, it has
typically taken two years or more—in the interim, the agency can raise
objections to certain components of the application, request new data or

further analysis of existing data, visit the sites where supporting studies were conducted, and conduct multiple reviews of the information submitted. An FDA review team generally includes experts in the fields of chemistry, pharmacology, medicine, statistics, and microbiology, all of whom apply their special expertise to analyzing the data. In deciding whether or not to approve a drug, the FDA never demands proof of absolute safety; the goal is a favorable balance between the risk of a drug and its potential benefit.

DRUG APPROVAL

Once a drug is approved, it can be put on the pharmacy shelves as soon as the sponsor is able to produce and distribute it. The whole process—from the time a drug enters clinical trials until it is approved—typically takes about eight years.

Appendix C

THE CHALLENGE TO THE AZT PATENT

BURROUGHS WELLCOME FILED its first American patent for AZT on September 17, 1985, and got approval from the U.S. Department of Commerce's Patent and Trademark Office nearly 2½ years later, after several rejections. From then on, the company had a seventeen-year exclusive monopoly that prevented anyone else from selling the drug.

The extortionate price that BW initially placed on AZT, coupled with its insistent efforts to minimize the involvement of government scientists in its development, turned patients, and later scientists, against the company. Eventually their anger unleashed a chain of events, documented elsewhere in this book, that resulted in a series of suits and countersuits to wrest the lucrative AZT patent from Burroughs Wellcome. Two Canadian companies were the first to challenge the patent in court, making their move in December 1990. Then, in March 1991, the Public Citizen Litigation Group formally filed its suit. Barr Labs's effort to have the government named coinventor came two months later.

The evidence unearthed so far supports both the patent challenge and other possible legal claims against BW in the future, based on the contentions that AZT treatment was not the sole invention of the Burroughs Wellcome Company, and that Burroughs Wellcome's application failed to satisfy three requirements of U.S. patent law—utility, non-obviousness, and novelty—as well as the duty of candor.

WAS AZT THE SOLE INVENTION OF BURROUGHS WELLCOME?

What the Law Says: A central doctrine of patent law is that every inventor be named in the application. To be coinventors—and thus to share a patent—parties need not prove that they have worked together, or at the same time, or even that they contributed equally to the claim. Rather, the law considers a party to be a coinventor when each one has contributed substantially to a step in the inventive process. The federal court has ruled that "one must be able to say that without his contribution to the final conception, it would have been less—less efficient, less simple, less economical, less some-thing of benefit."

How Burroughs Wellcome Stands Accused: Burroughs Wellcome chose to ignore this well-known requirement, submitting its patent request without naming a single collaborating government or academic scientist. The patent application strongly implied that BW was solely responsible for developing AZT as a treatment against AIDS. The omission of that crucial detail has become an important justification for challenging the patent's legality.

Perhaps to avoid charges of deliberate deceit, BW used vague language in its patent application, leaving open to question who actually performed the described experiments. Rather than using, for example, the words "we discovered," "we believe," or "our invention," the application used such phrases as "it has now been discovered," "it is believed," and "this invention." Nonetheless, the company began early to lay the groundwork for its claim to exclusive ownership of AZT.

Long before AIDS, when AZT was thought to hold promise as a cancer treatment, laboratory and animal tests had produced considerable information on the drug. Government researchers have said that this earlier data allowed clinical development of the compound to proceed quickly. But Burroughs Wellcome claimed in its 1988 annual report that "the fact that zidovudine had been synthesized as a possible anti-cancer agent years before had no bearing on the amount of time, effort, and money required for our investigation of its antiviral properties."

T. E. Haigler, BW's president at the time, also talked about the company's long-term involvement with AIDS research, calling it a natural extension of previous antiviral research. At hearings held by Congressman Henry Waxman in March 1987, and repeatedly at other public forums, Haigler kept underplaying the contributions made by the National Cancer Institute and Duke University and implying that all credit for the drug's availability rested with Burroughs Wellcome.

Sam Broder, head of the National Cancer Institute, fervently disagreed with Haigler's assessment and resented his efforts to steal the credit. In letters first sent privately to the company, and later made public, Broder repeatedly reminded Burroughs Wellcome that the development of AZT would not have occurred without the substantial commitment of government technology, resources, and personnel. He was especially irritated because BW had wreaked such havoc in his own lab by its eleventh-hour refusal to work with live AIDS virus. In a March 1987 letter to David Barry, BW's vice-president of research, Broder even suggested that the company was jeopardizing the government's ability to engage in joint ventures with the private sector. "In creating a possible record for lack of government involvement in the development of AZT before the Congress, you have greatly complicated our collaborative arrangements," wrote Broder.

Even as Burroughs Wellcome tried to pretend it had done all the footwork needed to develop AZT, letters were going back and forth between Sandra Lehrman, a senior research scientist in BW's Virology Department, and Sam Broder, attesting to their ongoing cooperation.

Lehrman wrote to Broder in October 1984: "I'm looking forward to a potentially productive and exciting collaboration."

And in March 1985 she wrote: "I feel our present collaboration and commitment to support future investigations has great potential for developing effective therapies for patients with AIDS."

Again in August: "Thanks for the continued commitment of your time and that of your clinical and research staffs in this collaborative effort to discover and develop drugs."

With the patent challenge now in court, the Lehrman-Broder correspondence will surely become one of the pivotal exhibits presented to illustrate just how closely BW worked with the government.

DID BURROUGHS WELLCOME DEMONSTRATE THE UTILITY AND NOVELTY OF AZT?

What the Law Says: American patent law requires applicants to demonstrate the "utility" and "novelty" of an invention. The goal is to prevent a company from filing a mountain of applications on the long-shot chance that one compound will someday prove useful. Or, as the Supreme Court has written in *Brenner* v. *Manson:* "A patent is not a hunting license. It is not a reward for the search, but compensation for its successful conclusion." To obtain a drug patent, an application must prove utility by providing the data to document a company's claims.

How Burroughs Wellcome Stands Accused: Burroughs Wellcome actually filed its first patent applications in England in March and May 1985, the latter four months before it filed in the United States. Because British patent law does not have the utility requirement, "prophetic" claims filed in the hope of a payoff are permissible. At the time of its first English patent application, utility had not been established; the company had done nothing more than repeat earlier animal testing. BW was hunting, having been

tipped off by previous research as to where the chemical herd might lie and
eager to forestall other claims to inventorship.

Laboratory testing was under way, however, and during the spring of
1985, NCI, Duke, and BW scientists jointly wrote an abstract documenting
the results of the test-tube experiments. Their abstract was presented at a
major scientific conference in October 1985, known as the Interscience Conference on Antimicrobial Agents and Chemotherapy (ICAAC), and published in fuller form that month in the *Proceedings of the National Academy
of Science*. The full-length article emphasized that the value of AZT in
humans was far from proven. "The activity of an agent against viruses
in-vitro does not ensure that the agent will be clinically useful in treating
viral diseases," wrote the authors. Other scientists were saying much the
same thing at the time.

Why did BW coauthor an article suggesting that lab findings on AZT could
not necessarily be transferred to patients while also submitting a patent
application that made bold claims about AZT's effectiveness? Most likely, it
was because BW did not want to alert its NCI and Duke collaborators that
it was filing a patent.

BW also did not want the patent office to know much about the ongoing
collaborations because that could have jeopardized its claim to sole inventorship and novelty. Also for that reason, its American application used the date
of the British patent filing as its priority filing date in the United States, and
preliminary results of the Phase I trials, which had been under way since
July 1985, were not disclosed.

However, BW's plan to hide the ongoing Phase I study initially backfired.
In January 1986 its first application was rejected, partly because it failed to
demonstrate utility. According to the patent office, the claim that AZT was
useful against HIV was "considered an incredible one at this time," and
adequate documentation to support it had not been provided.

Was AZT Obvious?

What the Law Says: In order to win a patent, the law requires that a drug's
effectiveness be "non-obvious." The legal test of obviousness is whether
knowledgeable observers believe a drug works before a patent is filed.
Almost always, such knowledge is derived from previously published findings.

How Burroughs Wellcome Stands Accused: Ironically, while BW's first
American patent application was rejected in part because utility had not
been proven, it was also turned down on the grounds that AZT's described

biological properties were obvious, given the work of earlier research. BW had dashed to file its American patent application before the October 1985 ICAAC proceedings were published, fearing the proceedings would render the invention obvious and thus unpatentable. BW presumably thought that when it filed its U.S. patent application in September, it had two weeks to spare before the publication date.

However, unknown to the company, the abstract had actually been published six weeks ahead of schedule and was mailed out to nearly 8,000 ICAAC members in late August.

When BW filed its British patent in March, AZT was a reasonable but unproven drug worthy of further study. But by the September patent application date in the U.S., AZT was the *only* obvious drug, at least in the eyes of the 8,000 ICAAC members who had seen the abstract.

DID BURROUGHS WELLCOME FULFILL ITS DUTY OF CANDOR?

What the Law Says: The law requires that a "duty of candor" be fulfilled when a patent application is filed. It is not enough to refrain from deceptive assertions; an application must also include all relevant information, even if it is detrimental. Certainly, one of the prime requirements of candor is that the application name all its coinventors.

How Burroughs Wellcome Stands Accused: BW's application gave the distinct impression that the company was alone in its discovery. After the patent office rejected the company's claims as obvious, BW wrote in rebuttal: "It is quite apparent that the NIH and others skilled in the art have been searching for a drug that will work, all apparently with little success to date."

Given the close working relationship with NCI and Duke, this was a direct misrepresentation. Why did BW lawyers respond to the patent office in such a misleading fashion? In all likelihood, because the company failed to disclose the information to its own lawyers. The violation of the duty of candor could be the final nail in the coffin of the patent's legitimacy.

THE PATENT GO-AHEAD

Despite major concerns about inventorship, utility, novelty, obviousness, and candor, Burroughs Wellcome's patent was finally approved in February 1988, after several tries.

How did this remarkable accomplishment take place? The reasons for the patent office's change of heart remain suspiciously unclear; only a thorough legal investigation will answer the question. For now, it is known that key documents likely to explain the shift in thinking at the patent office are missing, and there are hints that political pressures were brought to bear.

While the multitude of legal battles move through the courts, Burroughs Wellcome retains control of the AZT patent. Five years after the drug was approved, more than a billion dollars have poured into the coffers of Burroughs Wellcome. And still the black gold flows.

SOURCES

A NOTE ON SOURCES

Against the Odds is based on more than fifty personal interviews and thousands of pages of published and unpublished documents.

Crucial source material for this book came from congressional hearings. New York congressman Ted Weiss, chairman of the Human Resources and Intergovernmental Relations Subcommittee, Committee on Government Operations; California congressman Henry Waxman, chairman of the Subcommittee on Health and the Environment, Committee on Energy and Commerce; and Massachusetts senator Ted Kennedy, Committee on Labor and Human Resources, have taken the lead in spotlighting AIDS-related issues. Their offices provided us with transcripts of numerous hearings.

Transcripts of Food and Drug Administration (FDA) Advisory Committee meetings, held to debate the merits of AZT, aerosolized pentamidine, ganciclovir, ddI, parallel track and other major policy initiatives, were made available through Freedom of Information Act (FOIA) requests to the FDA. Also of value were transcripts of hearings held in 1989 and 1990 by the National Committee to Review Current Procedures for Approval of New Drugs for Cancer and AIDS (the Lasagna Committee) and the voluminous documentation collected by the Advisory Committee on the Food and Drug Administration (the Edwards Committee), which released its final report issued in May 1991. Other government documents were provided by the National Cancer Institute (NCI), the National Institute of Allergy and Infectious Diseases (NIAID), and the Food and Drug Administration.

Articles from the lay press—especially the *New York Times,* the *Wall Street Journal,* the *Washington Post,* and the *San Francisco Chronicle*—and from the medical literature—especially the *New England Journal of Medicine,* the *Journal of the American Medical Association, The Lancet, Nature,* and *Science*—were other vital sources of information. Specific articles are generally cited in the references that follow only where quotes were used,

273

an especially detailed analysis of an event was supplied, or a pivotal study was published.

The Documentation of AIDS Issues and Research Foundation, a San Francisco-based organization that is attempting to archive AIDS-related materials, and the Citizens Commission on AIDS, empaneled in New York City between 1987 and 1991 to stimulate more private sector involvement in AIDS-related issues, generously opened their files to us.

Unpublished memos and reports from ACT-UP's Treatment and Data Committee in New York provided crucial insights into the activists' perspective, as did a number of AIDS-related newsletters, including *AIDS Treatment News*, published by John James; *PI Perspective*, published by Project Inform; *Underground Notes*, published by the PWA Health Group; and *GMHC Treatment Newsletter*, published by the Gay Men's Health Crisis.

INTERVIEWS

Unless otherwise indicated, the quoted remarks in this book were obtained directly from in-person or telephone interviews. In a few instances, direct quotes were re-created from the recollections of those we interviewed.

The following is a complete list of interviews, many of which were taped and transcribed:

Donald Abrams, M.D., associate professor of clinical medicine, University of California, San Francisco; executive director, County Community Consortium, San Francisco, Calif.

John Arras, Ph.D., associate professor of bioethics, Department of Epidemiology and Social Medicine, Albert Einstein College of Medicine/Montefiore Medical Center, Bronx, N.Y.

Ron Baker, editor, *Bulletin of Experimental Treatments for AIDS*, San Francisco, Calif.

David Barr, attorney, formerly with Lambda Legal Defense, now with Gay Men's Health Crisis and ACT UP, New York, N.Y.

Terry Beswick, president, Community Research Alliance, San Francisco, Calif.

Bernard Bihari, M.D., former medical director, Community Research Initiative, New York, N.Y.

Marty Bleckman, Terry Sutton's roommate, San Francisco, Calif.

Dani Bolognesi, M.D., director, Duke Center for AIDS Research, Duke University Medical Center, Durham, N.C.

Paul Boneberg, executive director, Mobilization Against AIDS, San Francisco, Calif.

Sam Broder, M.D., director, National Cancer Institute, Bethesda, Md.

Pat Christen, executive director, San Francisco AIDS Foundation, San Francisco, Calif.

Ellen Cooper, M.D., former director, Antivirals Division, Center for Drug Evaluation and Research, FDA, Rockville, Md.

Michael Davis, law professor, Cleveland State University; expert on U.S. patent law, Cleveland, Ohio.

Martin Delaney, executive director, Project Inform, San Francisco, Calif.

Vincent DeVita, Jr., M.D., physician-in-chief, Memorial Sloan-Kettering Cancer Institute, New York, N.Y.; former director, National Cancer Institute, Bethesda, Md.

Lawrence Deyton, M.D., assistant director, Community Clinical Research, NIAID, Bethesda, Md.

Jim Eigo, member, AIDS Treatment and Data Committee, ACT UP, New York, N.Y.

Anthony Fauci, M.D., director, NIAID, Bethesda, Md.

Judith Feinberg, M.D., Johns Hopkins Medical School; former medical officer, Division of AIDS, NIAID, Bethesda, Md.

Morgan Fine, member, ACT UP, San Francisco, Calif.

Stuart Fisher, public relations executive, Geto & DeMilly, New York, N.Y.

Patsy Fleming, professional staff member, Human Resources and Intergovernmental Relations Subcommittee of the Committee on Government Operations, U.S. House of Representatives, Washington, D.C.

James M. Foster, consultant, Lyphomed; member, San Francisco Health Commission, San Francisco, Calif. Now deceased.

Gerald Friedland, M.D., director, AIDS Program, professor of medicine and epidemiology and public health, Yale University School of Medicine, New Haven, Conn.

Margaret Hamburg, M.D., commissioner, New York City Department of Health, New York, N.Y.; former assistant director, NIAID, Bethesda, Md.

Mark Harrington, member, AIDS Treatment and Data Committee, ACT UP, New York, N.Y.

Derek Hodel, executive director, PWA Health Group, New York, N.Y.

Robert Holzman, M.D., associate professor, New York University Medical Center, New York, N.Y.

Daniel Hoth, M.D., director, Division of AIDS, NIAID, Bethesda, Md.

John James, editor, *AIDS Treatment News,* San Francisco, Calif.

Robert Klein, M.D., associate professor, Department of Medicine and Department of Epidemiology and Social Medicine, Albert Einstein College of Medicine/Montefiore Medical Center, Bronx, N.Y.

Larry Kramer, co-founder, Gay Men's Health Crisis; co-founder, ACT UP, New York, N.Y.

Larry Krasnoff, former director, Biostatistics Division, Montefiore Medical Center, Bronx, N.Y.

Mathilde Krim, Ph.D., founding chairperson, American Foundation for AIDS Research, New York, N.Y.

Jay Lipner, attorney and activist, New York, N.Y. Now deceased.

Pierre Ludington, executive director, American Association of Physicians for Human Rights, San Francisco, Calif.

Jean McGuire, former director, AIDS Action Council, Washington, D.C.

Abbey Meyers, executive director, National Organization of Rare Disorders, New Fairfield, Conn.

Hiroaki Mitsuya, M.D., Ph.D., chief, Experimental Retrovirology Section, Medicine Branch, National Cancer Institute, Bethesda, Md.

Lynne M. Mofenson, M.D., Associate Branch Chief for Clinical Research, Pediatric, Adolescent and Maternal AIDS Branch, National Institute of Child Health and Human Development, NIH, Bethesda, Md.

A. Bruce Montgomery, M.D., AIDS researcher and Lyphomed consultant, San Francisco, Calif.

Andrew Moss, Ph.D., associate adjunct professor, Department of Epidemiology and Biostatistics, San Francisco General Hospital, San Francisco, Calif.

Russell Radley, director, Design Industries Foundation for AIDS, New York, N.Y.

Michelle Rolland, member, ACT UP, San Francisco, Calif.

Barbara A. Ryan, health care analyst, Prudential Bache, New York, N.Y.

Peter Staley, ACT UP, New York, N.Y.

Barbara Starrett, M.D., physician in private practice, New York, N.Y.

Brad Stone, acting director, Press Relations Staff, FDA, Rockville, Md.

Rick Storrs, staff, Documentation of AIDS Issues and Research Foundation, San Francisco, Calif.

Brian Tambi, president and chief executive officer, Fujisawa Pharmaceutical Company, formerly Lyphomed and now a subsidiary of Fujisawa of Japan.

Lewin Usilton, board chairman, Healing Alternatives Foundation, San Francisco, Calif.

Robert Veatch, director, Kennedy Institute of Ethics, Georgetown University, Washington, D.C.

Paul Volberding, M.D., chief, AIDS Program and Clinical Oncology, San Francisco General Hospital, San Francisco, Calif.

Hetty A. Waskin, M.D., Duke University Medical Center, Durham, N.C. Formerly with the Centers for Disease Control, Atlanta, Ga.

Tim Westmoreland, counsel, Health and the Environment Subcommittee of the Committee on Energy and Commerce, U.S. House of Representatives, Washington, D.C.

Brian Wolfman, attorney, Public Citizen, Washington, D.C.

Beverly Zakarian, president, Cancer Patients Action Alliance, Brooklyn, N.Y.

INTRODUCTION

The Reagan Administration's initial responses to AIDS are described in *The Federal Response to AIDS,* a congressional report by the Subcommittee on Human Resources and Intergovernmental Relations, House Committee on Government Operations, 98th Congr., 1st sess., 1983, and in *Review of the Public Health Service's Response to AIDS* (OTA-TM-H-24), a report by the Office of Technology Assessment, 1983. Three key books on the same subject are by Dennis Altman, *AIDS in the Mind of America* (Garden City, N.Y.: Anchor Press, 1986); Randy Shilts, *And the Band Played On: Politics, People and the AIDS Epidemic* (New York: St. Martin's Press, 1987); and Sandra Panem, *The AIDS Bureaucracy* (Cambridge, Mass.: Harvard University Press, 1988). See also Peter S. Arno and Karyn Feiden, "Ignoring the Epidemic: How the Reagan Administration Failed on AIDS," *Health/PAC Bulletin* 17 (1986): 7–11.

1: UNLIKELY HEROES

Larry Kramer wrote about "the time bomb" in *New York Native,* September 6, 1981. Robert Chesley's letter appeared in *New York Native,* January 3, 1982.

Two early reports focused attention on unusual diseases that were eventually linked to AIDS. The occurrence of PCP in five gay men in Los Angeles was described by the Centers for Disease Control in, "Pneumocystis Pneumonia," *Morbidity and Mortality Weekly* 30 (1981): 305–8. Kaposi's sarcoma, now known to accompany infection with the human immunodeficiency virus (HIV), was described in "Rare Cancer Seen in 41 Homosexuals," *New York Times,* July 3, 1981.

Larry Kramer accused Ellen Cooper of "Nazi-like tactics" at a public forum of the International AIDS Conference, Montreal, June 1989.

2: A New Virus: The Search for Magic Bullets

Kimberly Bergalis's letter in which she vividly described the symptoms of AIDS was released by her family in June 1991 and published widely in the popular press.

Twelve French scientists published their findings about the discovery of a virus associated with AIDS in F. Barre-Sinoussi, J.C. Chermann, et al., "Isolation of a T-Lymphotropic Retrovirus from a Patient at Risk for Acquired Immune Deficiency Syndrome (AIDS)," *Science* 220 (1983): 868–71.

For more on the discovery of HIV and the subsequent controversy over its true discoverer, see: Robert Gallo and Luc Montagnier, "The Chronology of AIDS Research," *Nature* 326 (1987): 435–36; Robert Gallo and Luc Montagnier, "AIDS in 1988," *Scientific American* 259 (1988): 41–48; Robert Crewdson, "The Great AIDS Quest," *Chicago Tribune*, November 9, 1989; J.C. Chermann et al., *Nature* 351 (1991): 277–78; Robert Gallo, Letter to the Editor, *Nature* 351 (1991): 358; "Gallo vs. Montagnier?," *Nature* 351 (1991): 426; Robert Gallo, *Virus Hunting: AIDS, Cancer & the Human Retrovirus* (New York: Basic Books, 1991).

The science of AIDS—how HIV invades the host, the course of infection, possible approaches for disabling the virus and descriptions of specific AIDS drugs—is contained in Peter T. Cohen, Merle A. Sande, Paul A. Volberding, *The AIDS Knowledge Base: A Textbook on HIV Disease from the University of California, San Francisco and the San Francisco General Hospital* (Waltham, Mass.: Medical Publishing Group, 1990). The *Knowledge Base* is also available on-line through BRS Colleague. Another source of scientific information is the quarterly *AIDS/HIV Treatment Directory*, available from the American Foundation for AIDS Research in New York. The range of therapeutic interventions that might disable HIV are well described in Hiroaki Mitsuya, Robert Yarchoan, Samuel Broder, "Molecular Targets for AIDS Therapy," *Science* 249 (1990): 1533–44.

3: The FDA and the Public Interest

For a historical overview of the Food and Drug Administration and descriptions of its approach to investigational drugs, see: Peter Barton Hutt, "Investigations and Reports Respecting FDA Regulation on New Drugs (Parts I & II), *Clinical Pharmacology and Therapeutics* 33 (1983): 538–48; Ellen J.

Flannery, "Should It Be Easier or Harder to Use Unapproved Drugs and Devices?," *Hastings Center Report* (February 1986): 17–23; Robert E. Wittes, "Noninvestigational Uses of Investigational Drugs: Some Implications of FDA's Revised Regulations," *Journal of the National Cancer Institute* 80 (1988): 301–4; David A. Kessler, "The Regulation of Investigational Drugs," *New England Journal of Medicine* 320 (1989): 281–88; transcripts of the Institute of Medicine Roundtable for the Development of Drugs and Vaccines Against AIDS, "Expanding Access to Investigational Therapies," March 12, 1990.

The increase in the annual AIDS research budget of the National Institutes of Health from $5.5 million in 1982 to $807 million in 1991 is itemized in the *Budget of the United States—Fiscal Year 1991*, U.S. Executive Office of the President, Office of Management and Budget, U.S. Government Printing Office, 1990, and updated by the NIH budget office. Economic data is also contained in Philip R. Lee and Peter S. Arno, "Federal Response to the AIDS Epidemic," *Health Policy* 6 (1986): 259–67.

The FDA's legislative responsibilities, its budget, and its inadequate workspace are documented in the "Final Report of the Advisory Committee on the Food and Drug Administration" (the Edwards Committee), May 1991.

The agency's drug approval record—792 drugs in 1988, 465 in 1989, 229 in 1990, and 327 in 1991—was provided by the agency's public information office.

The FDA's need for 2,000 more employees was asserted in *Comprehensive Assessment of Staffing, Facilities, and Equipment Needed*, a report by the U.S. General Accounting Office, September 1990.

For background about the ethics of human research and anecdotes about some of the more outrageous studies conducted during this century, see: Ruth Macklin and Gerald Friedland, "AIDS Research: The Ethics of Clinical Trials," *Law, Medicine, and Health Care* 14 (1986): 5–6, 273–80; Henry K. Beecher, "Ethics and Clinical Research," *New England Journal of Medicine* 274 (1966): 1354–60; David Rothman, "Ethics and Human Experimentation: Henry Beecher Revisited," *New England Journal of Medicine* 317 (1987): 1195–99; Carol Levine, "Has AIDS Changed the Ethics of Human Subjects Research?," *Law, Medicine & Health Care* 10 (1988): 167–73.

David Rothman, a medical historian at Columbia University, wrote that "no one objected to experiments on impaired inmates. In fact, researchers with links to custodial institutions had an edge in securing grants," in "Ethics and Human Experimentation."

The notorious Tuskegee syphilis experiment is painstakingly documented in James H. Jones, *Bad Blood: The Tuskegee Syphilis Experiment* (New York: The Free Press/Macmillan, 1981).

The ethical framework in place today for conducting clinical trials was established by the National Commission for the Protection of Human Subjects of Biomedical and Behavioral Research, *The Belmont Report*, Department of Health, Education and Welfare, 1978.

The FDA's budget of $5.2 million in 1955 and $11 million in 1960 is noted in Milton Silverman and Philip R. Lee, *Pills, Profits, and Politics* (Berkeley, Calif.: University of California Press, 1974).

The impact of the Kefauver Amendments is described in John C. Krantz, "The Kefauver-Harris Amendment After Sixteen Years," *Military Medicine* 143 (1978): 883 and in Louis Lasagna, "Congress, the FDA, and New Drug Development: Before and After 1962," *Perspectives in Biology and Medicine* 32 (1989): 322–43.

The number of Americans who used thalidomide on an experimental basis is provided in David Rothman and Harold Edgar, "New Rules for New Drugs: The Challenge of AIDS to the Regulatory Process," *The Milbank Quarterly* 68 (1990): 111–42.

The patient who protested his lack of access to experimental drugs, saying "It is as if I am in a disabled airplane, speeding downward out of control . . . ," was quoted in Martin Delaney, "The Case for Patient Access to Experimental Therapy," *Journal of Infectious Diseases* 159 (1989): 416–19.

Sam Kazman wrote that the FDA should announce "it will no longer stand between AIDS sufferers and the medicines they seek" in an editorial in the *Washington Post*, July 10, 1989.

The controversial claim that half the drugs approved in the United States for marketing have severe side effects was made by the General Accounting Office, *FDA Drug Review: Post Approval Risks 1976–1985*, April 1990. FDA official Bob Temple called the report "garbage in, garbage out" as cited in Philip J. Hilts, "Dangers of Some New Drugs Go Undetected, Study Says," *New York Times*, May 26, 1990.

Rothman and Edgar wrote of the irony that "sick gay men, abandoned by a President who refused publicly to acknowledge their disease, provided the shock troops to move forward his administration's deregulatory drug control program," in "New Rules for New Drugs."

Scam AIDS therapies were described by Marian Segal, "Defrauding the Desperate: Quackery and AIDS," *FDA Consumer* (1987): 20.

4: The AZT Breakthrough

Some of the events leading to the development of AZT were described in letters written by Sam Broder, now director of the National Cancer Institute, and officials of Burroughs Wellcome (BW) between October 1984 and December 1985, and were obtained via FOIA requests to NCI. Sam Broder, Hiroaki Mitsuya, also an NCI scientist, and Dani Bolognesi, a Duke University scientist involved in the early development of AZT, corroborated this information and provided further details in interviews. Another key government document was a memo from James B. Wyngaarden, director of the National Institutes of Health, to Robert E. Winsdom, assistant secretary for health, "History of Public Health Service Actions on Azidothymidine," February 4, 1987. The annual reports of the Burroughs Wellcome Company provide a different slant on AZT's development, as do Linda J. Wastila and Louis Lasagna, "The History of Zidovudine (AZT)," *Journal of Clinical Research and Pharmacoepidemiology* 4 (1990): 25–37.

The $250,000 cost of raising a lab to the P-3 level of safety is noted in the *Report of the Presidential Commission on the Human Immunodeficiency Virus Epidemic*, Washington, D.C., June 24, 1988.

Jerome Horwitz, the Detroit cancer researcher who first synthesized AZT, published his findings in Jerome P. Horwitz, J. Chua, et al., "The Monomesylats of 1-(2'-Deoxy-b-D-Lyxofuranosyl) Thymine," *Journal of Organic Chemistry* 29 (1964): 2076–78.

The first Phase I study to suggest AZT's value against HIV was Robert Yarchoan, Kent J. Weinhold, et al., "Administration of 3'-Azido-3'-Deoxythymidine, an Inhibitor of HTLV-III/LAV Replication, to Patients with AIDS or AIDS-Related Complex," *The Lancet* 1 (1986): 575–80. The Phase II results that established AZT's effectiveness were published as Margaret A. Fischl, Douglas D. Richman, et al., "The Efficacy of Azidothymidine (AZT) in the Treatment of Patients with AIDS and AIDS-Related Complex," *New England Journal of Medicine* 317 (1987): 185–91.

The recommendation to approve AZT on the basis of the Phase II AZT trials, and the debate preceding that decision, came at the FDA's Anti-Infective Drugs Advisory Committee meeting, January 16, 1987.

Janet Mitchell, chief of perinatology at Harlem Hospital, said "the concept that good research, pure research, is color-blind begs the issue . . ." before the Institute of Medicine's Committee to Study the AIDS Research Program of the National Institutes of Health, Washington, D.C., December 5, 1989.

5: PLACEBOS AND PROFITEERING

For an excellent discussion of the ethics of AIDS clinical trials see Carol Levine, Nancy Dubler, and Robert Levine, "Building a New Consensus: Ethical Principles and Policies for Clinical Research on HIV/AIDS," *IRB: A Review of Human Subjects Research* 13 (1991): 1–17. The debate over placebos is more specifically explored in Sissela Bok, "The Ethics of Giving Placebos," *Scientific American* 231 (1974): 17–23; Louis Lasagna, "Placebos and Controlled Trials Under Attack," *European Journal of Clinical Pharmacology* 15 (1979): 373–4; Robert J. Levine, "The Apparent Incompatibility Between Informed Consent and Placebo-Controlled Clinical Trials," *Clinical Pharmacology Therapeutics* (September 1987): 247–49. The activist perspective on placebo trials in AIDS is discussed in "Placebos: Time to Say No," *PI Perspective* 5 (1988): 1–4. New approaches to AIDS trial designs, developed partly in response to activist concerns about the ethics of traditional methods, are described in David P. Byar, David A. Schoenfeld, et al., "Design Considerations for AIDS Trials," *New England Journal of Medicine* 323 (1990): 1343–48.

The prolonged survival rate of patients taking AZT is documented in Richard Moore, Julia Hidalgo, et al., "Zidovudine and the Natural History of the Acquired Immunodeficiency Syndrome," *New England Journal of Medicine* 324 (1991): 1412–16. The effects of AZT in minority populations is documented in: Stephen Lagakos, Margaret A. Fischl, et al., "Effects of Zidovudine Therapy in Minority and Other Subpopulations with Early HIV Infection," *Journal of the American Medical Association* 266 (1991): 2709–12; and in Philippa J. Easterbrook, Jeanne C. Keruly, et al., "Racial and Ethnic Differences in Outcome in Zidovudine-Treated Patients with Advanced HIV Disease," *Journal of the American Medical Association* 266 (1991): 2713–18.

The recommendation not to take AZT—"AZT is not a cure for AIDS. . . . *Do not take, prescribe, or recommend AZT.*"—appeared in the *New York Native,* June 1, 1987.

T. E. Haigler, the former president of Burroughs Wellcome, described the company's research efforts and was grilled on the price of AZT during Congressman Henry Waxman's hearings, "AIDS Issues (Part I): Cost and Availability of AZT," Subcommittee on Health and the Environment, House Committee on Energy and Commerce, 100th Cong., 1st sess., 1987.

The Center for the Study of Drug Development, Tufts University, estimates the cost of developing a new drug to be $231 million; see: Joseph A. DiMasi, Ronald W. Hansen, et al., "Cost of Innovation in the Pharmaceutical Industry," *Journal of Health Economics* 10 (1991): 107–42. A study being prepared for Congress by the Office of Technology Assessment suggests that true costs are considerably lower, according to Milt Freudenheim, "Costs of Drug Research Seen as Overestimated," *New York Times,* April 30, 1991.

The first article to document the effectiveness of AZT against HIV in the test tube was Hiroaki Mitsuya, Kent J. Weinhold, et al., "3'-Azido-3'-Deoxythymidine (BW A509U): An Antiviral Agent That Inhibits the Infectivity and Cytopathic Effect of Human T-Lymphotropic Virus Type III/Lymphadenopathy-Associated Virus in Vitro," *Proceedings of the National Academy of Sciences* 82 (1985): 7096–7100.

Sam Broder wrote a letter to David Barry, BW's vice-president of research, to clarify the National Cancer Institute's contribution to AZT's development and to blast the company for its public posturing, March 19, 1987.

AZT sales figures from 1987 to 1991 were derived from Wellcome PLC's annual report, financial year ending August 31, 1991, London, England.

6: THE RISE OF THE AIDS UNDERGROUND

The techniques for smuggling ribavirin and isoprinosine into the United States from Mexico are outlined in "Federally Unapproved Medication for Treatment of AIDS: How to Get Them, How to Bring Them Home, How to Use Them," distributed by Project Inform, San Francisco, November 1986.

The letter suggesting that AL-721, a promising drug derived from egg yolks, might inhibit the AIDS virus appeared in Prem. S. Sarin, Robert Gallo, et al., "Effects of a Novel Compound (AL-721) on HTLV-III Infectivity in Vitro," *New England Journal of Medicine* 313 (1985): 1289–90. The rise in Ethigen's stock value soon afterward is documented in Marcia Barinage, "Controversial AIDS Drug for U.S. Market," *Nature* 332 (1988): 475. The continued delays in getting AL-721 tested led John James to call the drug "victim to a public policy nightmare" in *AIDS Treatment News*, April 4, 1987.

The history and operation of the People with AIDS Health Group, the New York City buyers' club, were described in interviews with the club's executive director, Derek Hodel. The operation of the Healing Alternatives Foundation (HAF), a San Francisco buyers' club, was described in interviews with Lewin Usilton, HAF board chairman, and other HAF staff.

A useful background on the science of unapproved AIDS therapies, including isoprinosine, AL-721, and dextran sulfate, and the underground efforts to obtain them, appears in Donald Abrams, "Alternative Therapies," in *Information on AIDS and HIV Infection and Disease: Monographs for Physicians and Other Health Care Workers* (Chicago: American Medical Association Press, 1989).

7: ACTIVISM, ACT UP, AND DEXTRAN SULFATE

Scientists set off a flurry of underground activity by suggesting that dextran sulfate was effective against HIV, letter by R. Ueno and S. Kuno, "Dextran

Sulfate, a Potent Anti-HIV Agent in Vitro Having Synergism with Zidovudine," *The Lancet* 1 (1987): 1379.

The underground network established to import dextran sulfate from Japan and the later demonstrations against Kowa Pharmaceuticals, one of the drug's manufacturers, were described in interviews with Martin Delaney, director of Project Inform, and Peter Staley, mastermind of many of ACT-UP's more theatrical protests.

The anonymous letter warning Donald Abrams, a leading AIDS researcher at San Francisco General Hospital, that cheating was taking place in his dextran sulfate trial is reprinted in Donald Abrams, "Alternative Therapies," in *Information on AIDS and HIV Infection and Disease: Monographs for Physicians and Other Health Care Workers* (Chicago: American Medical Association Press, 1989).

Larry Kramer called Tony Fauci, director of the National Institute for Allergy and Infectious Disease, a "monster" in an open letter, *Village Voice*, May 31, 1988 and said that everyone running "the AIDS show . . . is second-rate," at the Boston Lesbian and Gay Town Meeting, June 9, 1987. Kramer's call for terrorism at the Sixth International AIDS Conference in San Francisco was quoted in "A Call to Riot," *Outweek*, March 14, 1990.

Larry Kramer delivered the speech that launched ACT UP at the Lesbian and Gay Community Center, in New York, March 10, 1987; the speech is reprinted in *Reports from the Holocaust* (New York: St. Martin's Press, 1989). Although the definitive history of ACT UP has yet to be written, an illustrated record of its public protests is contained in Douglas Crimp, with Adam Roston, *AIDS Demographics* (Seattle: Bay Press, 1990). ACT UP's work is also described in David Handelman, "ACT UP In Anger," *Rolling Stone*, March 5, 1990, and Paul Taylor, "AIDS Guerillas," *New York Magazine*, November 12, 1990.

Former FDA Commissioner Frank Young announced a policy to allow people to import a three-month supply of unapproved pharmaceuticals for personal use at the National Lesbian and Gay Health Conference, in Boston, July 23, 1988. Young told a reporter that day, "I am not going to be the commissioner that robs them of hope," *New York Times*, July 24, 1988.

The Johns Hopkins University clinical trial that dampened enthusiasm for dextran sulfate is Kevin J. Lorentsen, Craig W. Hendrix, et al., "Dextran Sulfate Is Poorly Absorbed After Oral Administration," *Annals of Internal Medicine* 111 (1989): 561–66.

8: THE PENTAMIDINE SAGA

Robert Mony, an HIV-infected writer, described the symptoms of *Pneumocystis carinii* pneumonia (PCP) before a meeting of the FDA's Anti-Infective

Drugs Advisory Committee, May 1, 1989. Michael Callen, an AIDS activist, described the neglect of PCP research as a "scandal of unspeakable magnitude" and complained that "world-famous Ryan White did not know about the importance of PCP prophylaxis" at the same meeting.

For data on the costs of treating PCP and other AIDS-related conditions, see: Peter S. Arno and Jesse Green, "The Economics of AIDS," *The AIDS Knowledge Base*, ed. Peter T. Cohen, Merle A. Sande, Paul A. Volberding, et al. (Waltham, Mass.: Medical Publishing Group, 1990); Anne A. Scitovsky, Mary Cline, et al., "Medical Care Costs of Patients with AIDS in San Francisco," *Journal of the American Medical Association* 256 (1986): 3103–6; George R. Seage, Stewart Landers, et al., "Medical Care Costs of AIDS in Massachusetts," *Journal of the American Medical Association* 256 (1986): 3107–9.

Long before AIDS, pentamidine and Bactrim had already demonstrated their effectiveness against *Pneumocystis carinii* pneumonia. For a history of PCP and the drugs used to treat or prevent it, see: K. A. Western, D. R. Perera, et al., "Pentamidine Isethionate in the Treatment of *Pneumocystis Carinii* Pneumonia," *Annals of Internal Medicine* 73 (1970): 695–702; W. T. Hughs, P. C. McNobb, et al., "Efficacy of Trimethoprim and Sulfamethoxazole (Bactrim) in the Prevention and Treatment of *Pneumocystis Carinii* Pneumonitis," *Journal of Infectious Disease* 128 (1973): 607–11; W. T. Hughes, S. Kuhn, et al., "Successful Chemoprophylaxis for *Pneumocystis Carinii* Pneumonitis," *New England Journal of Medicine* 297 (1977): 1419–26.

The Centers for Disease Control's efforts to supply physicians with pentamidine and to find a manufacturer willing to produce it was described in interviews with Hetty A. Waskin, formerly with the CDC, and Abbey Myers, executive director of the National Organization for Rare Disorders (NORD) in New Fairfield, Connecticut.

In 1978, Lyphomed had monthly losses of $50,000 on sales that hovered around $1 million, according to Milt Freudenheim, "Lyphomed Sought by Fujisawa," *New York Times*, August 22, 1989.

The Orphan Drug Act, which provides financial incentives to pharmaceutical companies to conduct research on rare diseases, is Public Law 97-414. The history and objectives of the act are analyzed by Carolyn H. Asbury, *Orphan Drugs: Medical vs. Market Value* (Lexington, Mass.: Lexington Books, 1985); Naomi Siegel, "The Development of AZT: A Case Study of the Orphan Drug Act," Master's thesis, University of North Carolina, 1989; Carolyn H. Asbury, "The Orphan Drug Act: The First Seven Years," *Journal of the American Medical Association* 265 (1991): 893–97.

As of October 28, 1991, the FDA had granted orphan drug status to 473 drugs and approved 69 orphan drugs for marketing, according to Abbey Myers.

Donald Armstrong, chief of infectious diseases, Memorial Sloan-Kettering Cancer Center, described aerosol pentamidine's prophylactic properties against PCP in rats in "Aerosol Pentamidine," *Annals of Internal Medicine* 109 (1988): 852–54.

The struggle between NIAID and NCI for control of AIDS research is documented in an internal NIAID memo, "Background Information: Items for November 26 Meeting with Vince DeVita," November 24, 1986. Vince DeVita, then director of NCI, and Peggy Hamburg, then special assistant to Tony Fauci, corroborated and supplemented this information in follow-up interviews.

By 1991, 47 percent of NIAID's $400-million budget was devoted to AIDS research, according to *AIDS-Related Issues: How Has Federal Research on AIDS/HIV Disease Contributed to Other Fields?*, Office of Technology Assessment, U.S. Congress, April 1990.

The timetable that shows how aerosolized pentamidine trials were repeatedly delayed was supplied by NIAID on June 17, 1988, in response to a request by Congressman Henry Waxman.

Tony Fauci tried to explain the delay in testing aerosolized pentamidine, but eventually admitted he would try to secure the drug "on the street" if he had had a bout of PCP, at hearings held by Congressman Ted Weiss, "Therapeutic Drugs for AIDS: Development, Testing, and Availability," Subcommittee on Human Resources and Intergovernmental Relations, House Committee on Government Operations, 100th Cong., 2nd sess., April 28–29, 1988.

9: LOOSENING THE REGULATORY LEASH

General background about the Treatment IND innovation is provided in Grace Powers Monaco, J. D. Gottlieb, et al., "Treatment INDs: Research for Hire?," *Journal of the American Medical Association* 258 (1987): 3296–97; Frank E. Young, John A. Norris, Joseph A. Levitt, "The FDA's New Procedures for the Use of Investigational Drugs in Treatment," *Journal of the American Medical Association* 259 (1988): 2267–70; and Jeanne C. Conerly, "The IND Rewrite and the OMB: Business as Usual at the FDA?," *Columbia Journal of Law and Social Problems* 34 (1988): 1–30.

The Treatment IND initiative was called "a giant step for the sick and dying" in a *Wall Street Journal* editorial, March 13, 1987. The initiative was also said to "mark the end of an era when people with AIDS were forced to visit clandestine clinics," according to Lisa M. Krieger, *San Francisco Examiner,* April 12, 1987.

Congressman Ted Weiss expressed reservations about the Treatment IND and quoted from internal Office of Management and Budget documents to suggest that efforts were afoot to weaken the regulatory process in "FDA Proposals to Ease Restrictions on the Use and Sale of Experimental Drugs," Subcommittee on Human Resources and Intergovernmental Relations, House Committee on Government Operations, 100th Cong., 1st sess., April 29, 1987.

The small suramin study that showed promise was published by Sam Broder, Robert Yarchoan, et al., "Effects of Suramin on HTLV-III/LAV Infection Presenting as Kaposi's Sarcoma or AIDS-Related Complex: Clinical Pharmacology and Suppression of Virus Replication in Vivo," *The Lancet* 2 (1985): 627–30. After several patients died on Phase II suramin trials, researchers said the drug should be abandoned in Lawrence D. Kaplan, Peter R. Wolfe, et al., "Lack of Response to Suramin in Patients with AIDS and AIDS-Related Complex," *The American Journal of Medicine* 82 (1987): 615–20.

The final Treatment IND rule was published in the Federal Register, 52 FR 19466, May 22, 1987. Despite the surrounding controversy, Treatment IND was not "the lead paragraph in the obituary of the FDA," according to David Rothman and Harold Edgar, "New Rules for New Drugs: The Challenge of AIDS to the Regulatory Process," *The Milbank Quarterly* 68 (1990): 111–42.

Project Inform's Martin Delaney was quoted as calling FDA regulator Ellen Cooper "rigid and adamant in her beliefs" in *New York Times,* August 19, 1988. Delaney described his confrontation with Cooper in an interview.

Ted Weiss challenged the restrictive criteria imposed on the trimetrexate Treatment IND at his hearings, "Therapeutic Drugs for AIDS: Development, Testing, and Availability," Subcommittee on Human Resources and Intergovernmental Relations, House Committee on Government Operations, 100th Cong., 2nd sess., April 28–29, 1988. Further information about the distribution of trimetrexate and the effort to broaden the use of Treatment IND was obtained in interviews with Ellen Cooper, and with activists Jay Lipner, Martin Delaney, Jim Eigo, and David Barr.

New FDA procedures, informally known as Sub-Part E regulations and intended to expedite drug development and evaluation, were published as "Investigational New Drug, Antibiotic and Biological Drug Product Regulations; Procedures for Drugs Intended to Treat Life-Threatening and Severely Debilitating Illnesses," *Federal Register*, 53 FR 41523, October 21, 1988. At first, activists doubted that real change had taken place and the National Gay and Lesbian Task Force called the new regulations "a preelection gambit" according to Charles Marwick, "FDA Seeks Swifter Approval of Drugs for Some Life Threatening or Debilitating Diseases," *Journal of the American Medical Association* 260 (1988): 2976. ACT UP claimed the new regulations showed that "the 1988 Republican campaign wants to have an AIDS feather in its rather tattered cap," in its unpublished, but widely distributed, *FDA Action Handbook*, September 21, 1988.

10: Grassroots Trials Come of Age: Activists Seizing Control

The origins, philosophy, and growth of community-based drug testing were derived in part from interviews with Mathilde Krim, founding chair, American Foundation for AIDS Research (AmFAR); Bernard Bihari, former medical director, Community Research Initiative (CRI); Donald Abrams, executive director, County Community Consortium (CCC); and Carol Levine, executive director, Citizens Commission on AIDS. For further background about community trials, see: "Conference Proceedings, *Organizing Community-based Clinical Trials: Models for the AIDS Epidemic*," cosponsored by CRI and CCC, Columbia University, New York City, July 7–9, 1989. CRI's evolution is also described in a funding proposal to NIAID, "Contract Application of Community Research Initiative in Response to NIH-NIAID-AIDSP-89-II," Stage II, April 1989. CCC's history was traced by Abrams in his presentation before the National Commission on AIDS, Washington, D.C., May 8, 1990.

Nathaniel Pier claimed that current drug research "has not produced the goods" in "The Emperor Has No Clothes: Notes on Drug Testing and Access," *AIDS Patient Care* (February 1989): 2–5.

Joseph Sonnabend, one of CRI's founders, may have been right about the value of isoprinosine, according to C. Pedersen, E. Sandstrom, et al., "The Efficacy of Inosine Pranobex in Preventing the Acquired Immunodeficiency Syndrome in Patients with Human Immunodeficiency Virus Infection," *New England Journal of Medicine* 322 (1990): 1757–63. An accompanying editorial by FDA scientists, including Ellen Cooper, questioned the value of the study.

Margaret Fischl's controversial placebo-controlled Bactrim trial was published as M. A. Fischl, G. M. Dickinson, et al., "Safety and Efficacy of Sulfamethoxazole and Trimethoprim Chemoprophylaxis for *Pneumocystis*

Carinii Pneumonia," *Journal of the American Medical Association* 259 (1988): 1185–89.

Robert Mony, Michael Callen, David Feigal, and Ellen Cooper commented on aerosolized pentamidine at the FDA's Anti-Infective Drugs Advisory Committee meeting, May 1, 1989.

The long-delayed PCP prophylaxis recommendations issued by the National Institutes of Health were published by the Centers for Disease Control, "Guidelines for Prophylaxis Against *Pneumocystis Carinii* Pneumonia for Persons Infected with Human Immunodeficiency Virus," *Morbidity and Mortality Weekly Report* (June 16, 1989): 38.

The County Community Consortium's landmark trial, which led to the approval of aerosolized pentamidine, was published as Gifford S. Leoung, David W. Feigal, et al., "Aerosolized Pentamidine for Prophylaxis Against *Pneumocystis Carinii* Pneumonia: The San Francisco Community Prophylaxis Trial," *New England Journal of Medicine* 323 (1990): 769–75.

The failure to involve community-based physicians in AIDS drug research was an "underutilization of valuable resources," according to the *Report of the Presidential Commission on the Human Immunodeficiency Virus Epidemic,* June 24, 1988.

Health Secretary Louis Sullivan announced the establishment of eighteen community-based trial sites under NIAID's jurisdiction in a press release, October 5, 1989. For more details, see "Community Programs for Clinical Research on AIDS," *Background,* Community Clinical Research Section, Division of AIDS, NIAID, October/November 1989. The ongoing community trials funded by AmFAR are described in *AmFAR Report,* its periodic newsletter.

CRI issued a bitter press release when NIAID rejected its application, "NIAID Plays Politics with AIDS Funding: Punishes CRI–New York for Its Pioneering Role in Creating Alternative Approaches to AIDS Treatment Research," October 5, 1989. CRI also requested a debriefing letter and NIAID responded with "Request for Debriefing Under RFP NIH-NIAID-AIDSP-89-11: Community Programs for Clinical Research on AIDS," October 26, 1989. CRI criticized that debriefing in a fifteen-page rebuttal, November 30, 1989.

11: BUSINESS AS USUAL: THE PATENTING AND PRICING OF AZT

The meeting between Mark Harrington, Peter Staley, and David Barry, Burroughs Wellcome's vice-president of research, was described in an interview with Harrington.

ACT UP's invasion of BW's corporate headquarters in North Carolina was described in interviews with Peter Staley, who provided the blow-by-blow description re-created here, as well as in press accounts.

ACTG Protocol 016, which showed that AZT was effective in patients with early symptoms of HIV infection, was described in Margaret A. Fischl, Douglas D. Richman, et al., "The Efficacy of Azidothymidine (AZT) in the Treatment of Patients with AIDS and AIDS-Related Complex: A Double-Blind, Placebo-Controlled Trial," *New England Journal of Medicine* 317 (1987): 185–91.

Preliminary results of ACTG Protocol 019, which demonstrated that AZT could stave off symptoms of infection in HIV-positive people, were announced at a press conference, August 17, 1989. The dramatic rise in Burroughs Wellcome's stock price the following day and stock analyst Barbara Arzymanov's prediction of "quantum leap" stock price increases, were noted in Yann Tessier, "Wellcome Surges 32% in London as AZT Report Raises Prospect of Vast New Market for AIDS Drug," *Wall Street Journal*, August 21, 1989. The Protocol 019 study was finally published as Paul Volberding, Stephen Lagakos, et al., "Zidovudine in Asymptomatic Human Immunodeficiency Virus Infection: A Controlled Trial of Persons with Fewer than 500 CD4-Positive Cells per Cubic Millimeter," *New England Journal of Medicine* 322 (1990): 941–9.

The price of AZT was called "astoundingly high," in a lead editorial, "AZT's Inhuman Cost," the *New York Times*, August 28, 1989.

Congressman Henry Waxman wrote a private letter to T. E. Haigler, former BW president, in which he said, "the continued high price of the drug now appears to be an attempt to charge whatever patients, governments, and insurers can scrape together . . . ," September 7, 1989. Further pressure was put on BW when a coalition of sixteen AIDS organizations nationwide sent a memo to Haigler demanding that AZT's price be lowered, "Maximizing Access to Retrovir Through Price Reduction," August 31, 1989.

Jean McGuire of the AIDS Action Council described the meeting with BW, where no progress was made in efforts to reduce the cost of AZT, in an interview.

The invasion of the New York Stock Exchange was described in news accounts and interviews, with most specific details coming from Peter Staley.

T. E. Haigler wrote "had we been reluctant to direct the full force our research. . . . on this disease, there would have been no treatment for desperate patients . . ." in "Reduced Dosage Cuts Cost of AIDS Drug," letter, the *New York Times*, September 16, 1989. Hiroaki Mitsuya, Sam Broder, and others at the National Cancer Institute and Duke University responded to Haigler with their own letter, "Credit Government Scientists with Developing Anti-AIDS Drug," the *New York Times*, September 28, 1989.

Background about the legal challenge to Burroughs Wellcome's AZT patent came from letters requested under the Freedom of Information Act; court documents; BW's patent application; and extensive interviews with Michael Davis, law professor at Cleveland State University College of Law, and Brian Wolfman, an attorney with Public Citizen. Derek Hodel, executive director of PWA Health Group, provided further information in interviews. Bernadine Healy, director of the National Institutes of Health, backed Barr Lab's contention that NIH was entitled to share the AZT patent in a public statement May 28, 1991. More detailed citations about the patent challenge are provided in the source notes for Appendix C.

12: On the Defensive: Pentamidine Profits and a Corporation Under Siege

Lyphomed, the manufacturer of pentamidine, was a rising corporate star in the mid-1980s, "on everybody's can't miss, high-growth stock list," according to H. Lee Murphy, *Crain's Chicago Business,* May 30, 1988. Less than a year later, Lyphomed was faced with "lost customers, lost sales, lost image and lost shareholder value," according to the *Chicago Tribune*, May 15, 1989.

The FDA cited Lyphomed for forty-four "significant violations" of good manufacturing practices in a regulatory letter, November 13, 1987. Other regulatory conflicts with the FDA are outlined in Securities and Exchange Commission Form 10-Q, Commission file number 0-11280, quarter ended September 30, 1988.

The price hikes that brought pentamidine to $99.45 by August 1987 are documented in Robert Steinbrook, "Firm's Sharp Price Increase for AIDS Drug Attacked," *Los Angeles Times*, October 31, 1987, and Beverly Merz, "Aerosolized Pentamidine Promising in *Pneumocystis* Therapy, Prophylaxis," *Journal of American Medicine* 259 (1988): 3223–34.

Lyphomed's pricing policies were criticized by Congressman Ted Weiss and defended by Brian Tambi, then vice-president for corporate development, at hearings, "Therapeutic Drugs for AIDS: Development, Testing, and Availability," Subcommittee on Human Resources and Intergovernmental Relations, House Committee on Government Operations, 100th Cong., 2nd sess., April 28–29, 1988.

Lyphomed's stock prices in the mid-1980s, the company's estimated total sales and net losses, and the percentage of sales represented by pentamidine are documented by stock analyst, Barbara Ryan, *Bear Stearns Company Report on Lyphomed*, May 8, 1989. This information was corroborated in reports from the financial press and in a follow-up interview with Ryan.

Fujisawa's takeover of Lyphomed, related stockholder lawsuits, and the financial gains of John Kapoor, Lyphomed board chairman, are detailed in Securities and Exchange Commission document 14D-1, "Tender Offer to Purchase Lyphomed by Fujisawa Pursuant to Section 14(d)(1) and Amendment 13D Under the Securities and Exchange Act of 1934," September 8, 1989. Further financial and legal information about Lyphomed comes from Securities and Exchange Commission Form 10-Q, commission file number 0-11280, quarter ended September 30, 1989.

Lyphomed organized dog-and-pony shows in the fall of 1989, with the help of Geto & deMilley, a New York public-relations firm, to provide a spirited defense of its pentamidine pricing policies and to complain about the company's treatment by Congress, Fisons, and the AIDS underground. One such session, to which the authors were invited, is excerpted here.

Derek Hodel announced the PWA Health Group's intention to import cheaper pentamidine from England at a press conference, September 25, 1989, and provided further details in an interview. Brian Tambi's angry letter of protest to FDA Commissioner Frank Young, October 5, 1989, was furnished by Lyphomed. Jay Lipner's telephone call to Frank Young urging him not to issue an import alert for pentamidine was described by Lipner in an interview.

Edward Bernard, research associate at Memorial Sloan-Kettering, testified that if Fisons could not market its own version of aerosolized pentamidine, "we may be sentencing AIDS patients to less than the best available therapy . . .," before the Subcommittee on Health and the Environment, House Committee on Energy and Commerce, 101st Cong., 2nd sess., February 7, 1990.

For sales figures on "blockbuster orphan drugs," see: Deborah Erickson, "Big-Time Orphan: Human Growth Hormone Could be a Blockbuster," *Scientific American* (September 1990): 164–65; U.S. Department of Health and Human Services, Office of the Inspector General, "The Effect of the Interim Payment Rate for the Drug Epogen on Medicare Expenditures and Dialysis Facility Operations," September 4, 1990; Ann Gibbons, "Billion-Dollar Orphans: Prescription for Trouble," *Science* 248 (1990): 678–79; Carolyn Asbury, "The Orphan Drug Act: The First Seven Years," *Journal of the American Medical Association* 265 (1991): 893–97; and annual reports of Wellcome PLC, Amgen, and Genentech. Sales projections for pentamidine were extrapolated from *Bear Stearns Company Report on Lyphomed,* May 8, 1989.

Congressman Henry Waxman's amendments to the Orphan Drug Act, designed to curb excessive profits, were introduced as H.R. 4638, April 26, 1990. Hearings were held by Waxman's Health and the Environment Sub-committee, House Committee on Energy and Commerce, 101st Cong., 2nd sess., February 7, 1990. Opinion pieces on the Waxman amendments appeared in the *Wall Street Journal,* May 8, 1990. California congressman Pete Stark reintroduced the "Orphan Drug Windfall Profits Tax Cut of 1991," on October 10, 1991, and Kansas senator Nancy Kassebaum and Ohio senator Howard Metzenbaum introduced another reform bill on November 26, 1991.

For descriptions of the drug manufacturers lobby that sought to defeat the Orphan Drug Act Amendments of 1990, see: "Lyphomed Monopoly Could Be Affected by Drug Act Revision," *Wall Street Journal,* September 27, 1990; Ann Gibbons, "Orphan Drug Compromise Bush-Whacked," *Science* 250 (1990): 905; Jack Anderson, "Orphan Drug Veto Heats Up Lobbying," *Washington Post,* December 26, 1990. The role of the Competitiveness Council, chaired by Vice-President Dan Quayle, in President Bush's decision to veto the Orphan Drug Act, is described in an unpublished report, Christine Triano and Nancy Waltzman, "All the Vice President's Men: How the Quayle Council on Competitiveness Secretly Undermines Health, Safety, and Environmental Programs," September 1991. Abbey Meyers provided additional details about President Bush's veto.

Lyphomed's two-for-one sale to physicians, designed to boost pentamidine purchases, was described in an interoffice memorandum to the company's hospital sales managers, November 1, 1990. The memo was originally obtained by Derek Hodel and leaked to the press.

13: ABSENCE OF VISION: THE GANCICLOVIR SCANDAL

The compassionate-use program under which ganciclovir was distributed was described by public information officers at Syntex and Burroughs Wellcome.

The discussion of Syntex's initial application to market ganciclovir and its ultimate rejection were taken from transcripts of the FDA's Anti-Infective Drugs Advisory Committee meeting, October 26, 1987. Other details of the story were furnished by Jay Lipner, the AIDS activist, and Tony Fauci, NIAID director. Additional sources include Gina Kolata, "In AIDS, Virus Forces Choice Between Longer Life or Eyesight," *New York Times,* Decem-

ber 8, 1987, and Tim Kingston, "Justice Gone Blind: CMV Patients Fight for
Their Sight," *Coming Up*, February 1989.

The dinner meeting at which Tony Fauci told the activists "I'm one of the
best friends that you have" was held on December 17, 1987, and was
recorded by the activists.

The approval of ganciclovir was finally recommended, by a vote of 8–0
with one abstention, at the FDA's Anti-Infective Drugs Advisory Committee, May 2, 1989.

Peter Barton Hutt's comment that a "change in political climate" finally
led to the approval of ganciclovir was made at the annual meeting of the
American Public Health Association, New York City, September 30, 1990.

AIDS activist Terry Sutton's struggle to have foscarnet released to patients
who needed it was recounted in personal interviews with Michelle Rolland
and Marty Blechman, Sutton's close friends and fellow activists. Newspaper
accounts of the story include Lori Olazewski, "AIDS Protester Says He Faces
Blindness or an Earlier Death," *San Francisco Chronicle*, January 14, 1989,
and Dennis McMillan, "Activist Terry Sutton Dies of AIDS," *Bay Area
Reporter*, April 20, 1989.

ACT UP's Treatment and Data Committee asked the Swedish consulate
to pressure Astra to release foscarnet on a compassionate-use basis in a letter
dated May 15, 1989.

14: PARALLEL TRACK AND THE PROMISE OF DDI

The meeting called to flesh out the concept of parallel track, which is re-
created in some detail here, is culled from transcripts of the FDA's Anti-
Infective Drug Advisory Committee meeting, August 17, 1989. Other comments—including Martin Delaney's remark that "regulators today understand that we activists are not proponents of quackery . . ." and Jim Eigo's
denunciation of Treatment IND as "the same old lemon with tail-
fins . . ."—came in hearings called by Congressman Henry Waxman, Subcommittee on Health and the Environment, House Committee on Energy
and Commerce, 101st Cong., 1st sess., July 20, 1989.

Background information about parallel track and ddI comes in part from
interviews with Tony Fauci, director of NIAID, activists Jim Eigo and Jay
Lipner, Ellen Cooper, formerly of the FDA, and Sam Broder, director of
NCI.

The first study to show that ddI could inhibit HIV replication in the test
tube was published as Hiroaki Mitsuya and Samuel Broder, "Inhibition of
the in Vitro Infectivity and Cytopathic Effect of Human T-Lymphotropic

Virus Type III/Lymphadenopathy-Associated Virus (HTLV-III/LAV) by
2',3'-Dideoxynucleosides," *Proceedings of the National Academy of Science*
83 (1986): 1911–15. The Phase I results were published as Robert Yarchoan,
Hiroaki Mitsuya, et al., "In Vivo Activity Against HIV and Favorable Toxicity Profile of 2',3'-Dideoxyinosine," *Science* 245 (1989): 412–15.

The relative benefits and disadvantages of AZT and ddI are compared in
Hiroaki Mitsuya, Robert Yarchoan, et al., "Molecular Target for AIDS Therapy," *Science* 249 (1990): 1533–44.

The federal government granted Bristol-Myers the rights to develop and
market ddI in a licensing agreement, notable for the clause mandating
"reasonable pricing," signed in January 1988.

15: RESEARCH ON TRIAL: THE LIMITS OF THE GOVERNMENT SYSTEM

Information about the AIDS Clinical Trial Group (ACTG) comes partly from
interviews with Tony Fauci, Peggy Hamburg, Mathilde Krim, Gerald Friedland, Robert Klein, Martin Delaney, and Mark Harrington. Accounts of the
early efforts to build a research program—including the drugs that would be
studied and the enrollment problems that developed—came from NIAID's
AIDS Clinical Trials Advisory Group's *Final Report*, January 22, 1988 and
Institute of Medicine, *Report of a Workshop: The Potential Value of Research Consortia in the Development of Drugs and Vaccines Against HIV
Infection and AIDS*, Washington, D.C., 1989.

The late Barry Gingell vividly described the physical deterioration associated with AIDS at hearings called by Senator Ted Kennedy, Committee
on Labor and Human Resources, 100th Cong., 2nd sess., July 13, 1988.

The figure of $420 million sunk into the ACTG system by the end of 1991
was provided by the NIAID Budget Office, December 1991.

Thomas Merigan called NIAID's early efforts "the most powerful clinical
trials group for a single disease that this country has ever seen," personal
communication, December 1991.

Robert Bazell's article ("Medicine Show") on investigator-initiated research appeared in *New Republic*, January 22, 1990.

Barry Gingell's remarks, in which he complained that the ACTG restruc-
turing had accomplished little were read at Congressman Ted Weiss's hear-
ings by Kevin Armington of Gay Men's Health Crisis. See "Therapeutic
Drugs for AIDS: Development, Testing, and Availability," Subcommittee on
Human Resources and Intergovernmental Relations, House Committee on
Government Operations, 100th Cong., 2nd sess., April 28–29, 1988.

Paul Meier, vice-chair of a scientific panel evaluating the use of corticosteroids, revealed the professional jealousies that sometimes delay studies by quoting a colleague who held back findings that attributed a 50-percent reduction in mortality rates to steroids in Gina Kolata, "News of AIDS Therapy Gain Delayed Five Months by Agency," *New York Times,* November 14, 1990. The study was finally published as the National Institutes of Health–University of California Expert Panel for Corticosteroids as Adjunctive Therapy for Pneumocystis Pneumonia, "Consensus Statement on the Use of Corticosteroids as Adjunctive Therapy for Pneumocystis Pneumonia in the Acquired Immunodeficiency Syndrome," *New England Journal of Medicine* 323 (1990): 1500–1504.

The Peptide T story is recounted by Seth Holbein, "Peptide T and the AIDS Establishment," *Boston Magazine,* June 1990. Clinical studies of Peptide T sponsored by the National Institute of Mental Health are discussed in "New Drug Tested for Treatment of HIV, AIDS," *ADAMHA News,* May/June 1991.

The conflict-of-interest guidelines that would have limited researcher involvement with drug companies are contained in NIH Guide for Grants and Contracts, "Request for Comment on Proposed Guidelines for Policies on Conflict of Interest," September 15, 1989. Congressman Ted Weiss called the guidelines "strong minimum standards" and complained about loopholes in K.S. Jayaraman, "NIH Restricts University Links with Industry," *Nature* 341 (1989): 173.

The letter from the ACTG executive committee to Katherine Bick, who had drafted NIH's conflict-of-interest guidelines, was sent by Lawrence Corey, Donald Armstrong, M. Elaine Eyster, Margaret Fischl, Martin Hirsch, Gerald Medoff, Paul Volberding, and Catherine Wilfert, December 5, 1989.

The Pharmaceutical Manufacturers Association released a survey that indicated sixty-four different companies were studying medicines and vaccines for AIDS and AIDS-related conditions, *AIDS Medicines in Development,* October 11, 1991.

16: AIDS AND WOMEN, CHILDREN, AND MINORITIES

Chris Sandoval called the epidemic "an affirmative-action killer" at Ted Weiss's hearings, "The AIDS Crisis in Two American Cities," Subcommittee on Human Resources and Intergovernmental Relations, House Committee on Government Operations, 101th Cong., 1st sess., November 23, 1987.

The racial and ethnic composition of ACTG trial participants in 1990 is cited in James D. Eramo, D. Kirschenbaum, et al., "Women and Minorities

Have Less Access to AIDS Drug Trials," Seventh International Conference on AIDS, Florence, Italy, June 1991. The numbers of newly diagnosed AIDS cases in 1990 comes from Centers for Disease Control, "Update: Acquired Immunodeficiency Syndrome—United States, 1981–1990," *Morbidity and Mortality Weekly Report* 40 (1990): 357–69.

Mark Smith, a physician and researcher, formerly at Johns Hopkins School of Medicine, talked about the mistrust of minority people toward academic researchers at an Institute of Medicine Roundtable discussion, "Expanding Access to Investigational Therapies," March 13, 1990.

The exclusion of women from clinical trials is examined by NIH director Bernadine Healy, "The Yentyl Syndrome," *New England Journal of Medicine* 325 (1991): 275–77. Aspirin's value in protecting 22,000 male physicians against heart attacks was published by the Steering Committee of the Physicians Health Study Research Group, "Final Report on the Aspirin Component of the Ongoing Physicians' Health Study," *New England Journal of Medicine* 321 (1989): 129–35. Plans for a similar aspirin study in women, under NIH sponsorship, were reported by Lawrence K. Altman, "U.S. Plans Aspirin Study of Women," *New York Times*, July 29, 1991.

Sonia Singleton testified about the problems of enrolling in an appropriate clinical trial before the National AIDS Commission, Washington, D.C., May 7, 1990.

Nan Hunter of the American Civil Liberties Union criticized the exclusion of women from clinical trials at Ted Weiss's hearings, "Therapeutic Drugs for AIDS: Development, Testing, and Availability," Subcommittee on Human Resources and Intergovernmental Relations, House Committee on Government Operations, 100th Cong., 2nd sess., April 28–29, 1988.

Studies to investigate HIV transmission from mother to child were announced by NIAID, "Study of HIV-Infected Pregnant Women and Their Offspring to Begin," *Backgrounder*, March 8, 1991.

Taryn Lindhorst describes the "courtesy stigma" in "Women and AIDS: Scapegoats or a Social Problem?," *Affilia* 3 (1988): 51–59.

The man identified as Joe described the ordeals he faced in seeking treatment for his sixteen-month-old daughter at Ted Weiss's hearings, "Therapeutic Drugs for AIDS: Development, Testing, and Availability," Subcommittee on Human Resources and Intergovernmental Relations, House Committee on Government Operations, 100th Cong., 2nd sess., April 28–29, 1988.

The study design and results of ACTG Protocol 045, in which intravenous immunoglobulin was tested in children, were published by the National Institute of Child Health and Human Development Intravenous Immunoglobulin Study Group, "Intravenous Immune Globulin for the Prevention of Bacterial Infections in Children with Symptomatic Human Immunodeficiency Virus Infection," *New England Journal of Medicine* 325 (1991): 73–80.

Nicholas Rango talked of "therapeutic nihilism" at Weiss hearings, "Treatment and Care for Persons with HIV Infection and AIDS," Subcommittee on Human Resources and Intergovernmental Relations, House Committee on Government Operations, 101st Cong., 1st sess., July 28–August, 1, 1989.

The growth of AIDS among drug users compared to gay men is derived from Centers for Disease Control, "Update: Acquired Immunodeficiency Syndrome—United States, 1981–1990."

Wafaa El-Sadr, chief of infectious diseases at Harlem Hospital, said that excluding whole categories of sick people on the basis of color, sex, age, or behavior was "inappropriate social policy, bad public health practice, and poor science," at Ted Weiss's hearings, "Treatment and Care for Persons with HIV Infection and AIDS," Subcommittee on Human Resources and Intergovernmental Relations, House Committee on Government Operations, 101st Cong., 1st sess., July 28–August, 1, 1989.

17: THE ILLICIT COMPOUND Q TRIALS

Much of the information about Compound Q came from interviews with Martin Delaney and Ellen Cooper. Key press accounts included Frank Browning, "The Question of Q," in *In Health*, September/October 1990, and Gina Kolata, "Critics Fault Secret Effort to Test AIDS Drug," *New York Times*, September 19, 1989. Project Inform also described its decision to test Compound Q in a "Dear Concerned Friend" letter, July 18, 1989.

Results of Compound Q animal tests were published as Michael S. McGrath, Hin-Wing Yeung, et al., "GLQ-223: An Inhibitor of Human Immunodeficiency Virus Replication in Acutely and Chronically Infected Cells of Lymphocyte and Mononuclear Phagocyte Lineage," *Proceedings of the National Academy of Science* 86 (1989): 2844–48.

The FDA issued two Talk Papers to clarify its position on Project Inform's Compound Q trial—"FDA Okays Clinical Testing of GLQ-223," April 27, 1989, and "FDA Statement on Unauthorized AIDS Drug Study," June 28, 1989.

Martin Delaney defended his Compound Q trial while Arnold Relman, former editor of the *New England Journal of Medicine*, called the preliminary results "black magic," at the Sixth International Conference on AIDS, San Francisco, June 1990.

Studies under the auspices of San Francisco General Hospital and Project Inform were published in the same issue of the journal *AIDS*. The San Francisco General study was published as James O. Kahn, Lawrence D. Kaplan, et al., "The Safety and Pharmacokinetics of GLQ-223 in Subjects with AIDS and AIDS-Related Complex: A Phase I Study," *AIDS* 4 (1990): 1197–1204. The Project Inform study was published as Vera S. Byers, Alan S. Levin, et al., "A Phase I/II Study of Trichosanthin Treatment of HIV Disease," *AIDS* 4 (1990): 1189–96.

18: THE DDI MILESTONE

Gina Kolata's controversial article about ddI was "Innovative AIDS Drug Plan May Be Undermining Testing," *New York Times*, November 21, 1989. ACTG researcher Douglas Richman and Jerome Groopman were quoted in the same article. Her second provocative piece, "Odd Surge Found in Deaths of Those Taking AIDS Drug," *New York Times*, March 12, 1990, included the quote from ACTG researcher Thomas Chalmers. The letter of response by twenty-three community activists was published as "Don't Blame Drug Program for AIDS Deaths," *New York Times*, March 28, 1990.

The proposed parallel-track policy, including a request for comments, was published as "The Expanded Availability of Investigational New Drugs Through a Parallel Track Mechanism for People with AIDS and HIV-Related Diseases," *Federal Register*, May 21, 1990, 20856–60.

Martin Delaney wrote a private letter to FDA officials Ellen Cooper and Paul Beninger, in which he said ddI and ddC had already shown "reasonable proof of some degree of efficacy," and should be approved, August 16, 1990.

The FDA's intensive effort to get ddI approved and its novel methodology were described by scientists in the agency's antiviral division at the FDA's Anti-Infective Drugs Advisory Committee meeting, July 18–19, 1991. Remarks by FDA Commissioner David Kessler, Carl Peck, director of the Center for Drug Evaluation and Research, Donald Abrams, San Francisco General Hospital researcher, and Theodore Eicklhoff, of the University of Colorado at Denver, come from that meeting.

The number of patients enrolled in ddI clinical trials and in the expanded access program were obtained from a Bristol-Myers Squibb press release, "Videx (Didanosine): Its Discovery and Development," October 9, 1991.

19: CRASHING THE GATES: ACTIVISTS ENTER THE DRUG TESTING SYSTEM

Details of the activists' interactions with the AIDS Clinical Trial Group researchers were provided by Tony Fauci, Jim Eigo, Mark Harrington, and Larry Kramer. The response of many ACTG researchers to activist participation in their decision making was also reported in Jesse Dobson "Fear and Loathing in Bethesda," *San Francisco Sentinel*, April 26, 1990. Mark Harrington wrote that the Germans were more graceful about opening up the Berlin Wall than the ACTG researchers were about allowing activists into their meetings, "In the Belly of the Beast," *Outweek*, October 1989.

ACT-UP harshly criticized the accomplishment and priorities of the ACTG system in "A Critique of the AIDS Clinical Trials Group." ACTG scientists were given a preliminary draft of the report at their March 7, 1990, meeting and a final version at their May 1, 1990, meeting. Mark Harrington also critiqued the ACTG system in "Anatomy of a Disaster: Why Is Federal AIDS Research at a Standstill?," *The Village Voice*, March 13, 1990. NIAID countered with "NIAID Responds to ACT UP Allegations and Demands," May 16, 1990, and ACT UP produced a rebuttal, "ACT UP Responds to NIAID's Allegations and Evasions," May 21, 1990.

CONCLUSION

The warning to "hurry up—carefully" was made by Benjamin Freedman, "Nonvalidated Therapies and HIV Disease," *Hastings Center Report*, May/June 1989.

The *Wall Street Journal* criticized the FDA's advisory committee meeting's initial decision not to recommend tacrine's approval in "The AIDS Hoax," March 18, 1991. More sympathetic analyses of the issues involved were Gina Kolata, "Surprise in Delay of Alzheimer's Disease," *New York Times*, March 17, 1991, and Gina Kolata, "FDA Panel Approves Test Distribution of Alzheimer's Drug," *New York Times*, June 16, 1991.

Reporter Phil Hilts wrote that Tony Fauci had been given a "pass through the sea of anger" in "Despite Advocates' Anger at U.S., AIDS Research Chief Wins Respect," *New York Times*, September 4, 1990.

Beverly Zakarian, president of the Cancer Patients Action Alliance, described the emerging activist movement among cancer patients in an interview. The subject is also covered in Ora Baer, "FDA, Congress to Feel Political Pressure from Cancer Patients," *Oncology Times*, September 1990, and Jane Gross, "Turning Disease into Political Cause: First AIDS, and Now Breast Cancer," *New York Times*, January 7, 1991. Susan Love's Washington speech was excerpted in *Breast Cancer Action Newsletter* no. 6, June 1991.

The controversy over clozapine pricing was widely covered in the press, including Milt Freudenheim, "Maker of Schizophrenia Drug Bows to Pressure to Cut Costs," *New York Times,* December 6, 1990, and Ron Wislow, "Sandoz Sets Clozaril Price, Abandoning Combined Charge for Drug, Blood Tests," *Wall Street Journal,* January 15, 1991.

Hiroshi Nakajima, the director-general of the World Health Organization, estimates that between 30 and 40 million persons will be infected with HIV by the year 2000, according to *Wall Street Journal,* November 29, 1991.

APPENDIX B: HOW A CLINICAL TRIAL IS DESIGNED

The primer on clinical trials design is derived from: FDA, *From Test Tube to Patient: New Drug Development in the United States,* March 1990. See also Terra Ziportx, "The Food and Drug Administration: How Those Regulations Came to Be," *Medical News* 254 (October 1985): 2037–46 and David A. Kessler, "The Regulation of Investigational Drugs," *New England Journal of Medicine* 320 (1989): 281–88.

APPENDIX C: THE CHALLENGE TO THE AZT PATENT

Three general sources provided most of the documentation for the challenge to Burroughs Wellcome's AZT patent—letters received under the Freedom of Information Act, legal documents and personal interviews. The letters include a series dated October 1984 through December 1985 between Sandra Nusinoff Lehrman, senior research scientist at Burroughs Wellcome's Department of Virology, David Barry, then head of BW's Virology Department, and Sam Broder, then associate director of the Clinical Oncology Program, National Cancer Institute.

The court documents reviewed are: *People with AIDS Health Group et al.* v. *Burroughs Wellcome Co.,* filed in the United States District Court for the District of Columbia, March 18, 1991; *Burroughs Wellcome Co.* v. *Barr Laboratories, Inc.,* filed in United States District Court for the Eastern District of North Carolina, May 14, 1991; *Apotex Inc. and Novopharm Ltd.* v. *The Wellcome Foundation Limited,* filed in the Federal Court of Canada, Trial Division, December 5, 1990.

Insights into the AZT patent challenge also come from BW's patent applications, including: Patent and Trademarks Office, United States Department of Commerce, patent filed by J. Rideout et al., serial number 776899, September 17, 1985; BW's July 14, 1986 rebuttal to the Patent Office's rejections by BW's attorneys: J. Rideout et al., amendment remarks, July 1986. Also key were extensive interviews with Michael Davis, professor of law at Cleveland State University College of Law, and Brian Wolfman, an attorney with Public Citizen, who are attorneys for the plaintiffs in *People with AIDS Health Group et al.* v. *Burroughs Wellcome Co.* Additional information was obtained in interviews with Derek Hodel of PWA Health Group.

The concept that speculative or experimental utility is insufficient to support a patent application is contained in *Brenner* v. *Manson*, 383 U.S. 519, 16 L. Ed. 2d 69, 86 S. Ct. 1033, 148 U.S. P. Q. 689; 1966.

The abstract in which NCI, Duke University, and BW researchers first reported test tube results indicating AZT's effectiveness was presented at Interscience Conference on Antimicrobial Agents and Chemotherapy, October 19, 1985. The full article is Hiroaki Mitsuya, Kent J. Weinhold, et al., "3'-Azido-3'-Deoxythymidine (BW A509U): An Antiviral Agent That Inhibits the Infectivity and Cytopathic Effect of Human T-Lymphotropic Virus Type III/Lymphadenopathy-Associated Virus in Vitro," *Proceedings of the National Academy of Sciences* 82 (1985): 7096–7100.

BW denied that the earlier syntheses of AZT had a bearing on its own research in the annual report of Wellcome PLC, 1988.

INDEX

Abrams, Donald, 72, 113, 181, 223
  CCC and, 113–16, 123
Abrams, Robert, 104
Acetone, 65
ACLU (American Civil Liberties
  Union), 150
ACTG, *see* AIDS Clinical Trial Group
ACT UP (AIDS Coalition to Unleash
  Power), 61, 73–80, 122, 196
  birth of, 73–74, 75
  foscarnet and, 170–71
  ganciclovir and, 161, 164–65
  invasion of New York Stock
    Exchange, 134–37
  invasion of offices of BW, 127–30
  involvement inside drug-testing
    system, 225–35
  logo of, 75
  tactics of, 76–82, 108
  Treatment IND and, 107–9
  weekly meetings of, 75–76
Acquired Immune Deficiency
  Syndrome, *see* AIDS
Acyclovir, 38, 57
Affilia, 202
African sleeping sickness, 84, 99
Agnos, Art, 146
AIDS (journal), 214
AIDS (Acquired Immune Deficiency
  Syndrome):
  account of suffering from, 11–12, 187
  cause of, 14, 16
  changes in behavior due to, 7
  course of the disease, 16–17
  defined, 16, 200–201
  demographics of, 199, 205, 206, 233,
    243
  early passivity concerning, 6–7

first published reports on, 3–4
incubation period, 16
mandatory testing for, 11
naming of, 4
national strategy on, 5
statistics on, 1, 44, 199, 205, 206
vaccine for, 20–21
AIDS Action Council, 134, 135, 183
AIDS activists, 2, 6–9, 105, 237–38
  grassroots trials and, 110–24
  Hyatt Regency conference and,
    179–84
  involvement in drug research system,
    225–35, 238, 242–43
  *see also names of individuals and
    organizations*
AIDS Clinical Trial Group (ACTG), 91,
  93, 113, 122, 131, 163, 187, 263
  AIDS activists and, 225–35
  battle over focus of research, 192–93
  blacks and, 198–99
  children and, 202–5
  committee scoring and, 190, 194,
    196–97
  conflicts of interest and, 193–96
  criticism of, 186–97, 207–8, 242–43
  ddI and, 216–24
  directed research and, 190, 191
  drug users and, 205–6
  grassroots trials and, 123–24
  investigator-initiated research and,
    190–92
  Opportunistic Infection Committee,
    193
  parallel track and, 173, 174, 176–77,
    185
  Primary Infection Committee, 193,
    228, 235